Current Clinical Pathology

Series Editor
Antonio Giordano, Philadelphia, PA, USA

This series includes monographs dealing with important topics in surgical pathology, cytopathology hematology, and diagnostic laboratory medicine. It is aimed at practicing hospital based pathologists and their residents providing them with concise up-to- date reviews and state of the art summaries of current problems that these physicians may encounter in their daily practice of clinical pathology.

More information about this series at https://link.springer.com/bookseries/7632

Cardio-Oncology

Management of Toxicities in the Era of Immunotherapy

Antonio Russo • Nicola Maurea
Dimitrios Farmakis • Antonio Giordano
Editors

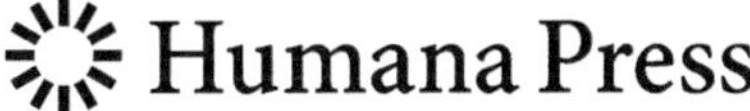 Humana Press

Editors
Antonio Russo
Department of Surgical, Oncological, and
Oral Sciences
University of Palermo
Palermo, Italy

Dimitrios Farmakis
University of Cyprus Medical School
Nicosia, Cyprus

Nicola Maurea
Istituto Nazionale Tumori IRCCS
Fondazione G. Pascale
Napoli, Italy

Antonio Giordano
Sbarro Institute for Cancer Research
& Molecular Medicine
Temple University
Philadelphia, PA, USA

ISSN 2197-781X ISSN 2197-7828 (electronic)
Current Clinical Pathology
ISBN 978-3-030-97746-7 ISBN 978-3-030-97744-3 (eBook)
https://doi.org/10.1007/978-3-030-97744-3

This Humana imprint is published by the registered company Springer Nature Switzerland AG
The registered company address is: Gewerbestrasse 11, 6330 Cham, Switzerland

Foreword

The field of cardio-oncology is evolving rapidly. Between old and novel oncological drugs, treatment-associated cardiotoxicity is a significant cause of morbidity and mortality in cancer survivors. With the development of novel and more effective therapies, such as immunotherapy, there is a higher risk of significant cardiac toxicities in oncological patients.

This book comprehensively covers all the aspects of cardio-oncology, with a particular emphasis on cardiotoxicities' management.

Moreover, this book is a study guide and a valuable tool for oncologists, cardiologists, and medical oncology residents, focusing on the mechanisms of immunotherapy-associated cardiotoxicity, risk factors, detection methods, and treatment. Knowledge of this type of toxicity among both cardiologists and oncologists is crucial for determining the scope of this problem and systematically formulating treatment strategies in the light of multidisciplinary teamwork.

I would like to congratulate Professors Antonio Russo, Nicola Maurea, Dimitrios Farmakis, and all their coworkers for the great effort and work.

Finally, my best wishes to the publishing team of Springer Nature for working diligently with the authors in bringing out such a unique textbook.

University of Palermo   Massimo Midiri, MD
Palermo, Italy

Preface

Clinical oncology is a rapidly evolving field. The achievements made during the last several decades empowered continuous improvements in clinical oncology's sphere of influence. Several targeted therapy and immunotherapy are changing the clinical landscape and the natural history of many tumors, impacting patients' survival.

Moreover, the main aim of this textbook was to highlight the importance of cross-fraternity discussions for better patient care, because of the necessity for a medical oncologist to discuss with other healthcare providers such as cardiologists the novel scenario of cardiotoxicity in the era of immunotherapy.

In this textbook, different specialists in the field have covered many aspects of the management of cardiac toxicities. The first chapters provide a comprehensive overview and background information on tumor biology and immunotherapy, while the remaining chapters include different aspects of cardiotoxicities' management, diagnosis, and treatments.

Furthermore, even while advances and approvals in oncology are at a fast pace, an oncology trainee needs to be aware, understand, and apply basic clinical methods, principles, and knowledge in daily practice, more so in resource-constrained settings. This textbook offers an invaluable, practice-oriented tool for medical students just beginning their clinical oncology studies, as well as medical oncology residents and young professionals.

In this light, I am confident that this book will provide a direction to students and oncology residents to think and act accordingly.

Palermo, Italy   Antonio Russo

Acknowledgments

I convey my sincere appreciation to the national and international faculty for their contributions to this book.

I would like to congratulate all the authors for writing such a much-needed book. I am deeply grateful to all the authors for accepting to make an incredible journey together, hoping to bring a valuable, practice-oriented tool for the future generation of healthcare professionals.

Lastly, I wholeheartedly would like to thank Springer Nature for its hard work in bringing this book to reality.

Antonio Russo

Contents

Contributors

Chiara Brando Department of Surgical, Oncological, and Oral Sciences, University of Palermo, Palermo, Italy

Maria Laura Canale Cardiology, Versilia Hospital, Azienda USL Toscana Nord Ovest - Lido di Camaiore (LU), Toscana, Italy

Ettore Capoluongo Dipartimento di Eccellenza in Medicina Molecolare e Biotecnologie Mediche, Università Federico II, Naples, Italy

DAI – Medicina di Laboratorio e Trasfusionale, Azienda Ospedaliera Universitaria Federico II, Naples, Italy

CEINGE – Biotecnologie Avanzate, Naples, Italy

Andreina Carbone National Cancer Institute, IRCCS Pascale, Naples, Italy

Giuseppe Curigliano Division of Early Drug Development for Innovative Therapies, European Institute of Oncology IRCCS, Milan, Italy

Department of Oncology and Hemato-Oncology, University of Milan, Milan, Italy

Daniela Di Lisi Cardiology Unit, University Hospital Paolo Giaccone, Palermo, Italy

Department of Health Promotion, Mother and Child Care, Internal Medicine and Medical Specialties (ProMISE), University of Palermo, Palermo, Italy

Dimitrios Farmakis University of Cyprus Medical School, Nicosia, Cyprus

Antonio Galvano Department of Surgical, Oncological, and Oral Sciences, University of Palermo, Palermo, Italy

Stefania Gori Medical Oncology, IRCCS Ospedale Sacro Cuore Don Calabria, Negrar di Valpolicella, Verona, Italy

Valerio Gristina Department of Surgical, Oncological, and Oral Sciences, University of Palermo, Palermo, Italy

Federica Iacono Department of Surgical, Oncological, and Oral Sciences, University of Palermo, Palermo, Italy

Lorena Incorvaia Department of Experimental Biomedicine and Clinical Neurosciences, School of Medicine, University of Palermo, Palermo, Italy

Alessandro Inno Medical Oncology, IRCCS Ospedale Sacro Cuore Don Calabria, Negrar di Valpolicella, Verona, Italy

Martina Iovine National Cancer Institute, IRCCS Pascale, Naples, Italy

Fabian Islas Cardiovascular Institute, San Carlo Hospital, Madrid, Spain

Maria La Mantia Department of Surgical, Oncological, and Oral Sciences, University of Palermo, Palermo, Italy

Chiara Lisanti Department of Surgical, Oncological, and Oral Sciences, University of Palermo, Palermo, Italy

Girolamo Manno Cardiology Unit, University Hospital Paolo Giaccone, Palermo, Italy

Department of Health Promotion, Mother and Child Care, Internal Medicine and Medical Specialties (ProMISE), University of Palermo, Palermo, Italy

Nicola Maurea Istituto Nazionale Tumori IRCCS Fondazione G. Pascale, Napoli, Italy

Stefania Morganti Division of Early Drug Development for Innovative Therapies, European Institute of Oncology IRCCS, Milan, Italy

Department of Oncology and Hemato-Oncology, University of Milan, Milan, Italy

Giuseppina Novo Cardiology Unit, University Hospital Paolo Giaccone, Palermo, Italy

Department of Health Promotion, Mother and Child Care, Internal Medicine and Medical Specialties (ProMISE), University of Palermo, Palermo, Italy

Vincenzo Quagliariello National Cancer Institute, IRCCS Pascale, Naples, Italy

Antonio Russo Department of Surgical, Oncological, and Oral Sciences, University of Palermo, Palermo, Italy

Paolo Tarantino Division of Early Drug Development for Innovative Therapies, European Institute of Oncology IRCCS, Milan, Italy

Department of Oncology and Hemato-Oncology, University of Milan, Milan, Italy

Paola Zagami Division of Early Drug Development for Innovative Therapies, European Institute of Oncology IRCCS, Milan, Italy

Department of Oncology and Hemato-Oncology, University of Milan, Milan, Italy

Background: Immunology and Cancer

Lorena Incorvaia, Valerio Gristina, Chiara Brando,
Maria La Mantia, and Antonio Russo

Over the past few decades, a growing body of evidence has progressively led to a better understanding of the interactions between tumor and immune cells, highlighting the key role of the immune system in suppressing the development and progression of cancers [1]. Several different therapeutic approaches boosting the body's natural defense have consistently reported durable responses in a wide range of cancer histotypes, showing that cancer immunotherapy is a promising and active treatment modality [2]. In addition to the encouraging activity, such immune-related approaches have been associated with manageable safety profiles that are somewhat different from traditional systemic or targeted cancer therapies [3]. The success of these therapies displays the importance of careful understanding of basic immunology for successful clinical translation in oncology [4, 5].

The capacity of the immune system to recognize and fight external offenses (such as antimicrobial agents) has been well established [6, 7]. The success of vaccines in preventing disease shows that the immune system has "host protective memory," represented by innate and adaptive immunity [6, 8]. Namely, while the innate immune system is capable of rapid response without immunological memory towards specific targets, adaptive immunity is based on B and T cells that allow the recognition of specific antigens that eventually trigger durable immune responses [6, 9]. In particular, B and T cells mediate the specific immunity producing the antibody and T-cell receptor (TCR) repertoire, respectively. In this vein, when specifically considering the interactions between cancer and immune cells, the immune

L. Incorvaia
Department of Experimental Biomedicine and Clinical Neurosciences, School of Medicine, University of Palermo, Palermo, Italy
e-mail: lorena.incorvaia@unipa.it

V. Gristina · C. Brando · M. La Mantia · A. Russo (✉)
Department of Surgical, Oncological, and Oral Sciences, University of Palermo, Palermo, Italy
e-mail: valerio.gristina@unipa.it; chiabra92@libero.it; maria.lamantia@unipa.it

A. Russo et al. (eds.), *Cardio-Oncology*, Current Clinical Pathology,
https://doi.org/10.1007/978-3-030-97744-3_1

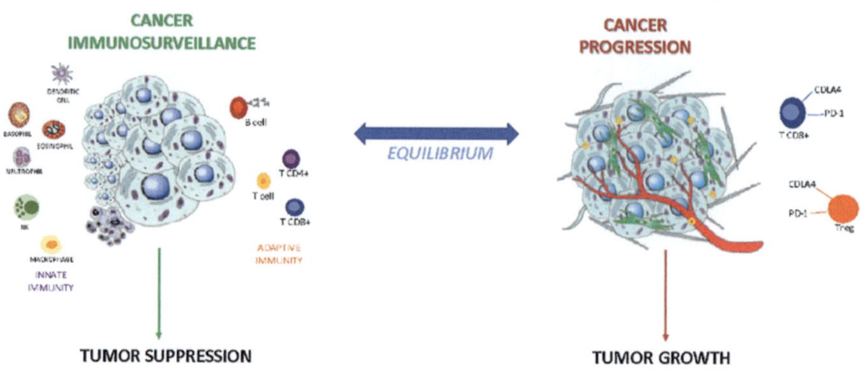

Fig. 1.1 The complex interplay between cancer and the immune TME

system seems to play a dual role in suppressing and promoting tumor progression, a process which is termed "cancer immunoediting" and consists of three phases: elimination, equilibrium, and escape [10, 11]. As such, emerging evidence suggests that tumors are composed not merely of neoplastic cells but also of the tumor microenvironment (TME), a milieu of different cell types including endothelial cells, several stromal cell types, and immune components [12] (Fig. 1.1).

In this fascinating scenario, a series of steps must be pursued to carry out an effective immune response against cancer. Accordingly, due to the genomic instability caused by the uncontrolled proliferation of cancer cells, a large number of neoantigen proteins are released into the bloodstream and then phagocytosed by macrophages and dendritic cells (antigen-presenting cells, APC), finally migrating through the draining lymphatic vessels towards regional lymph nodes [13]. Herein, neoantigens would be presented via the major histocompatibility complex (MHC)-TCR interaction to naive T cells [14, 15]. Moreover, the final naive T-cell activation requires other crucial co-stimulatory signals, represented by the ligation of the CD28 receptor (constitutively expressed on T cells) and the B7 superfamily proteins (B7.1 and B7.2, expressed on APCs), to finally promote the clonal expansion and differentiation in memory T cells, either tumor-specific (CD4+) or directly cytotoxic (CD8+) [16, 17].

Especially in advanced cancer stages, even if immune and cancer cells could coexist in a dynamic steady state, the persistence of this phenomenon may lead to the real exhaustion of tumor-specific T cells which become anergic undergoing a sort of functional paralysis and expressing inhibitory immune checkpoints on their surface to elude and suppress the immune response [18, 19]. The cytotoxic T-lymphocyte-associated antigen 4 (CTLA-4) and programmed death 1 (PD-1), expressed on the T cells surface, are immune checkpoints that trigger the inhibition of T-cell activity after binding to the respective ligands expressed on the tumor cell surface (CD 80/CD86 and PD-L1/PD-L2, respectively), thus playing a key role in the control of the antitumor immune response [20, 21]. Namely, after APCs present antigens to the naïve T cells, therefore leading to the final T-cell activation, CTLA-4 is upregulated, inhibiting the T-cell response in the priming phase (activation phase); even if the complex PD-1/PD-L1 interactions are also involved in this phase, the PD-1 receptor serves to inhibit the T-cell response in the effector phase (killing phase) [22].

In clinical practice, the most well-established specific immunotherapy for cancer is represented by monoclonal antibodies. Anti-CTLA-4 and anti-PD-1 antibodies bind to CTLA-4 and PD-1, turning off the inhibitory signal and thus enhancing the T-cell function in the lymph nodal and peripheral tissues, respectively [23, 24]. In this scenario, the complex interplay between cancer and the immune TME could crucially affect the outcome of immunotherapy while activating autoreactive T cells and resulting in a wide range of immune-related adverse events (irAEs) [25]. Even if rare and underreported in early clinical trials, ICI-associated cardiotoxicity emerged as a serious and life-threatening event that, unlike other irAEs involving differing organs, may be refractory to glucocorticoids [26].

References

 1. Mellman I, Coukos G, Dranoff G. Cancer immunotherapy comes of age. Nature. 2011;480(7378):480–9. https://doi.org/10.1038/nature10673.
 2. Mullard A. New checkpoint inhibitors ride the immunotherapy tsunami. Nat Rev Drug Discov. 2013;12, no. 7. England:489–92. https://doi.org/10.1038/nrd4066.
 3. Magee DE, et al. Adverse event profile for immunotherapy agents compared with chemotherapy in solid organ tumors: a systematic review and meta-analysis of randomized clinical trials. Ann Oncol Off J Eur Soc Med Oncol. 2020;31(1):50–60. https://doi.org/10.1016/j.annonc.2019.10.008.
 4. Russo A, et al. The molecular profiling of solid tumors by liquid biopsy: a position paper of the AIOM-SIAPEC-IAP-SIBioC-SIC-SIF Italian scientific societies. ESMO open. 2021;6(3):100164. https://doi.org/10.1016/j.esmoop.2021.100164.
 5. Passiglia F, et al. Is there any place for PD-1/CTLA-4 inhibitors combination in the first-line treatment of advanced NSCLC?-a trial-level meta-analysis in PD-L1 selected subgroups. Transl Lung Cancer Res. 2021;10(7):3106–19. https://doi.org/10.21037/tlcr-21-52.
 6. Weiner LM. Cancer immunology for the clinician. Clin Adv Hematol Oncol. 2015;13(5):299–306.
 7. Gristina V, et al. Is there any room for PD-1 inhibitors in combination with platinum-based chemotherapy as frontline treatment of extensive-stage small cell lung cancer? A systematic review and meta-analysis with indirect comparisons among subgroups and landmark survival analyses. Ther Adv Med Oncol. 2021;13:17588359211018018. https://doi.org/10.1177/17588359211018018.
 8. Russo A, et al. The tumor-agnostic treatment for patients with solid tumors: a position paper on behalf of the AIOM- SIAPEC/IAP-SIBioC-SIF Italian scientific societies. Crit Rev Oncol Hematol. 2021;165:103436. https://doi.org/10.1016/j.critrevonc.2021.103436.
 9. Incorvaia L, et al. Baseline plasma levels of soluble PD-1, PD-L1, and BTN3A1 predict response to nivolumab treatment in patients with metastatic renal cell carcinoma: a step toward a biomarker for therapeutic decisions. Onco Targets Ther. 2020;9(1):1832348. https://doi.org/10.1080/2162402X.2020.1832348.
10. Schreiber RD, Old LJ, Smyth MJ. Cancer immunoediting: integrating immunity's roles in cancer suppression and promotion. Science (80-). 2011;331(6024):1565–70. https://doi.org/10.1126/science.1203486.

11. Incorvaia L, et al. BRCA1/2 pathogenic variants in triple-negative versus luminal-like breast cancers: genotype-phenotype correlation in a cohort of 531 patients. Ther Adv Med Oncol. 2020;12:1758835920975326. https://doi.org/10.1177/1758835920975326.

12. Hu M, et al. Distinct epigenetic changes in the stromal cells of breast cancers. Nat Genet. 2005;37(8):899–905. https://doi.org/10.1038/ng1596.

13. Martin K, Schreiner J, Zippelius A. Modulation of APC function and anti-tumor immunity by anti-cancer drugs. Front Immunol. 2015;6:501. https://doi.org/10.3389/fimmu.2015.00501.

14. Attaf M, Legut M, Cole DK, Sewell AK. The T cell antigen receptor: the Swiss army knife of the immune system. Clin Exp Immunol. 2015;181(1):1–18. https://doi.org/10.1111/cei.12622.

15. Passiglia F, et al. PD-L1 expression as predictive biomarker in patients with NSCLC: a pooled analysis. Oncotarget. 2016;7(15):19738–47. https://doi.org/10.18632/oncotarget.7582.

16. Esensten JH, Helou YA, Chopra G, Weiss A, Bluestone JA. CD28 costimulation: from mechanism to therapy. Immunity. 2016;44(5):973–88. https://doi.org/10.1016/j.immuni.2016.04.020.

17. Passiglia F, et al. Looking for the best immune-checkpoint inhibitor in pre-treated NSCLC patients: an indirect comparison between nivolumab, pembrolizumab and atezolizumab. Int J Cancer. 2018; https://doi.org/10.1002/ijc.31136.

18. Farkona S, Diamandis EP, Blasutig IM. Cancer immunotherapy: the beginning of the end of cancer? BMC Med. 2016;14:73. https://doi.org/10.1186/s12916-016-0623-5.

19. Incorvaia L, et al. Challenges and advances for the treatment of renal cancer patients with brain metastases: from immunological background to upcoming clinical evidence on immune-checkpoint inhibitors. Crit Rev Oncol Hematol. 2021;163:103390. https://doi.org/10.1016/j.critrevonc.2021.103390.

20. Buchbinder EI, Desai A. CTLA-4 and PD-1 pathways: similarities, differences, and implications of their inhibition. Am J Clin Oncol. 2016;39(1):98–106. https://doi.org/10.1097/COC.0000000000000239.

21. Badalamenti G, et al. Role of tumor-infiltrating lymphocytes in patients with solid tumors: can a drop dig a stone? Cell Immunol. 2019;343:103753. https://doi.org/10.1016/j.cellimm.2018.01.013.

22. Galvano A, et al. The prognostic impact of tumor mutational burden (TMB) in the first-line management of advanced non-oncogene addicted non-small-cell lung cancer (NSCLC): a systematic review and meta-analysis of randomized controlled trials. ESMO Open. 2021;6(3) https://doi.org/10.1016/j.esmoop.2021.100124.

23. Incorvaia L, et al. Programmed death ligand 1 (PD-L1) as a predictive biomarker for Pembrolizumab therapy in patients with advanced non-small-cell lung cancer (NSCLC). Adv Ther. 2019; https://doi.org/10.1007/s12325-019-01057-7.

24. Seidel JA, Otsuka A, Kabashima K. Anti-PD-1 and anti-CTLA-4 therapies in cancer: mechanisms of action, efficacy, and limitations. Front Oncol. 2018;8:86. https://doi.org/10.3389/fonc.2018.00086.

25. Novo G, et al. Arterial stiffness: effects of anticancer drugs used for breast cancer women. Front Physiol. 2021;12:661464. https://doi.org/10.3389/fphys.2021.661464.

26. Passiglia F, et al. Monitoring blood biomarkers to predict nivolumab effectiveness in NSCLC patients. Ther Adv Med Oncol. 2019;11:1758835919839928. https://doi.org/10.1177/1758835919839928.

Available Immunotherapy Drugs in Oncology

2

Valerio Gristina, Federica Iacono, Chiara Lisanti, Maria La Mantia, and Antonio Galvano

Recently, the advent of immune-oncology (IO) represented a breakthrough in the evolving landscape of cancer therapeutics. Several clinical trials have shown the relevant value of programmed death 1 (PD-1), programmed death ligand-1 (PD-L1), and cytotoxic T-lymphocyte antigen 4 (CTLA-4) checkpoint inhibitors, leading to better progression-free survival (PFS) and overall survival (OS) compared with standard treatments. Moreover, immunotherapy is usually well-tolerated with manageable side effects and good quality of life (QoL) [1, 2]. The improved understanding of the tumor immune response and immune escape from the host's immune system has elucidated the therapeutic role of immunity in the genesis of cancer [3]. The immune system is recognized as an essential tool in cancer biology due to its effect on cancer growth, tumor development, and metastasis process [4]. Therefore, cancer therapeutic studies have been particularly focused on the immune system [5, 6]. There are different classifications of Food and Drug Administration (FDA)- and European Medicines Agency (EMA)-approved immunotherapy treatments, and they involve anti-PD-1 (nivolumab, pembrolizumab) and anti-PD-L1 (atezolizumab, durvalumab, avelumab) antibodies [7].

Table 2.1 summarizes the available immunotherapy drugs in oncology.

V. Gristina · F. Iacono · C. Lisanti · M. La Mantia · A. Galvano (✉)
Department of Surgical, Oncological, and Oral Sciences, University of Palermo, Palermo, Italy
e-mail: antonio.galvano@unipa.it

A. Russo et al. (eds.), *Cardio-Oncology*, Current Clinical Pathology,
https://doi.org/10.1007/978-3-030-97744-3_2

Table 2.1 Summary of the available immunotherapy drug in oncology

Drug	Drug target	Isotype	Indications
Pembrolizumab	Anti-PD-1	IgG4	Melanoma, NSCLC, HNSCC, UC, MSI-H, GC, CC, HCC, RCC, EC, ESCC, MSI-H/dMMR CRC, TNBC
Nivolumab	Anti-PD-1	IgG4	Melanoma, NSCLC, HNSCC, UC, MSI-H, GC, MPM, RCC, HCC, MSI-H/dMMR CRC, SCLC
Atezolizumab	Anti-PD-L1	IgG1	NSCLC, SCLC, TNBC, HCC, Melanoma, UC
Durvalumab	Anti-PD-L1	IgG1	NSCLC, SCLC, UC
Avelumab	Anti-PD-L1	IgG1	RCC, UC
Ipilimumab	Anti-CTLA-4	IgG1	Melanoma, NSCLC, RCC, MSI-H/dMMR CRC, MPM, HCC

Abbreviations: *NSCLC* non–small cell lung cancer, *HNSCC* head and neck squamous cell carcinoma, *UC* urothelial carcinoma, *MSI-H* microsatellite instability-high, *GC* gastric cancer, *CC* cervical cancer, *HCC* hepatocellular carcinoma, *RCC* renal cell carcinoma, *EC* endometrial cancer, *ESCC* esophagus cancer, *dMMR* mismatch repair deficient, *TNBC* triple-negative breast cancer, *MPM* malignant pleural mesothelioma, *SCLC* small-cell lung cancer

Anti-PD-1 Agents

Pembrolizumab

Pembrolizumab is an IgG4 fully humanized anti-PD-1 antibody, which binds to the PD-1 receptor and blocks its interaction with PD-L1 and PD-L2, leading to PD-1 pathway-mediated inhibition of the immune response [8, 9]. Pembrolizumab is approved for different cancer histotypes, such as small cell lung cancer (SCLC), head and neck squamous cell carcinoma (HNSCC), urothelial carcinoma, gastric cancer, esophageal cancer, cervical cancer, hepatocellular carcinoma, Merkel cell carcinoma, renal cell carcinoma, and endometrial carcinoma. Moreover, in 2017, FDA approved pembrolizumab for metastatic microsatellite instability-high (MSI-H) or mismatch repair-deficient (dMMR) tumors nonresponsive to prior treatment and for metastatic MSI-H or dMMR colorectal cancer progressed with a fluoropyrimidine, oxaliplatin, and irinotecan therapy [6, 10]. As mentioned above, pembrolizumab is currently approved for the treatment of patients with unresectable or metastatic melanoma and for the adjuvant treatment of patients with melanoma with involvement of lymph nodes after complete resection [11, 12]. The first approval by the FDA was in 2015 based on data from KEYNOTE-001 and KEYNOTE-002 [13–15]. Particularly, KEYNOTE-002 is a multicenter, randomized, active-controlled trial that investigated the efficacy of ipilimumab-refractory melanoma in 540 patients randomized to receive one of two doses of pembrolizumab (2 mg/kg and 10 mg/kg) or investigator's choice chemotherapy [13, 16]. The study demonstrated a statistically significant improvement in PFS (HR 0.57, 95% CI 0.45–0.73). Considering the KEYNOTE-006 results, which compared pembrolizumab to ipilimumab in the first or second line, pembrolizumab was approved for metastatic patients with untreated melanoma regardless of BRAF mutation [17, 18]. Indeed, this randomized open-label multicenter trial demonstrated an impressive OS benefit in favor of pembrolizumab (32.7 vs 15.9 months (HR 0.73 (95%CI 0.61–0.89)) and a statistically significant improvement in PFS for patients randomized to pembrolizumab as compared to ipilimumab [18, 19]. Recently, pembrolizumab was approved in the adjuvant setting due to the results of KEYNOTE-054, which randomized patients with resected stage IIIA-B-C melanoma to pembrolizumab or placebo [20]. In fact, the authors reported a statistically significant improvement in relapse-free survival (RFS) for patients randomized to the pembrolizumab arm. The risk of recurrence in the total population was 43% lower in the pembrolizumab group than in the placebo one. Additionally, in the overall intention-to-treat (ITT) population, the 18-month rate of recurrence-free survival was 71.4% for pembrolizumab vs. 53.2% for placebo, respectively [20].

Over the last decades, major progress in non–small cell lung cancer (NSCLC) treatment strategies was related to the advent of immunotherapy. Indeed, immunotherapy with anti-PD1 therapies extremely modified the treatment approach for locally advanced and metastatic NSCLC [21, 22]. Following the KEYNOTE-010 trial, pembrolizumab was approved as a second-line treatment for PDL-1 positive patients with advanced NSCLC who have progressed to a first-line treatment with chemotherapy [23, 24]. KEYNOTE-010 is a randomized phase II/III trial, which compared pembrolizumab with docetaxel in patients with a PD-L1 expression $\geq$of 1%. In the overall population, the OS was considerably longer for pembrolizumab: the median OS was 12.7 months with pembrolizumab and 8.5 months in the docetaxel arm. In 2016, pembrolizumab started to play an important role as a single agent in the first-line treatment of NSCLC, thanks to the KEYNOTE-024 trial which compared pembrolizumab to platinum-based chemotherapy [25, 26]. In fact, 305 patients with previously untreated advanced NSCLC, PD-L1 expression of $\geq$50%, and no sensitizing mutation of the epidermal growth factor receptor (*EGFR*) gene or translocation of the anaplastic lymphoma kinase (*ALK*) gene were randomized to receive either pembrolizumab or platinum-based chemotherapy. Pembrolizumab was associated with an improved response rate (RR) (44.8% vs. 27.8%) and median PFS (10.3 vs. 6.0 months, HR 0.5; 95% CI: 0.37–0.68) [25, 27]. Consequently, the FDA granted approval of pembrolizumab for naïve patients with metastatic NSCLC and no sensitive mutation with a PDL-1 $\geq$ 50%, becoming the new standard of care for the first-line treatment of this subset of patients. Thereafter, pembrolizumab was investigated in NSCLC patients with PD-L1 < 50%. Notably, the KEYNOTE-042 confirmed the superiority of pembrolizumab compared to chemotherapy in patients with high PD-L1 expression and showed similar outcomes in those with PD-L1 score of 1–49% [28]. Latterly, pembrolizumab has been investigated in KEYNOTE-189 in combination with chemotherapy in the front-line setting in adenocarcinoma, showing improvement in OS and PFS [29, 30]. The study compared pemetrexed and a platinum-based drug plus either 200 mg of pembrolizumab or placebo every 3 weeks for four cycles, followed by pembrolizumab or placebo for up to a total of 35 cycles plus pemetrexed maintenance therapy. Of note, although the greatest relative benefit was observed in the subgroup with a PD-L1 tumor proportion score of 50% or greater, the benefit of the pembrolizumab combination was observed in all subgroups, including those with a PD-L1 tumor proportion score of less than 1%. The PFS was 8.8 mo. (95% CI 7.6–9.2) with the combination vs 4.9 mo. (95% CI 4.7–5.5) for the standard arm. The HR for progression or death was 0.52 (95% CI 0.43–0.64) [30, 31]. Likewise, KEYNOTE-407 investigated the role of pembrolizumab plus chemotherapy for untreated patients with squamous histology, showing a statistically significant improvement in OS (15.9 vs 11.3 HR 0.64), PFS (6.4 vs 4.8 HR 0.56), and ORR (58% vs 35%) for patients randomized to pembrolizumab in combination with chemotherapy [26, 32].

Based on these trials, pembrolizumab was finally approved as first-line treatment for metastatic non-squamous NSCLC with no EGFR or ALK genomic tumor aberrations in combination with pemetrexed and platinum chemotherapy and as first-line treatment for patients with metastatic squamous NSCLC in combination with chemotherapy. Furthermore, the efficacy of pembrolizumab was investigated also in small-cell lung cancer (SCLC) in three trials: the phase 1b KEYNOTE-028, Cohort C1, and the phase II KEYNOTE-158, Cohort G. Based on these clinical trials, pembrolizumab was approved for the treatment of patients with SCLC who had progressed on/after chemotherapy and at least one other prior line of therapy. Noteworthy, a recent pooled analysis of patients from KEYNOTE-028 and KEYNOTE-158 showed a durable antitumor activity in a subset of patients with recurrent or metastatic SCLC who had previously been treated with two or more lines of therapy, regardless of PD-L1 expression. The analysis reported an ORR of 19.3% compared with 18.7% for the overall population in KEYNOTE-158, in which patients were enrolled irrespective of their PD-L1 status, and 33.3% for KEYNOTE-028, which enrolled only patients with PD-L1–positive tumors. Moreover, the analysis showed similar median OS and PFS (7.7 and 2.0 mo, respectively) in comparison with those from the overall populations (median OS was 9.7 and 8.7 months and median PFS was 1.9 and 2.0 mo for KEYNOTE-028 and KEYNOTE-158, respectively) [33, 34].

Before the era of ICIs, few treatment options were available for patients with metastatic urothelial carcinoma (UC) [35, 36]. Pembrolizumab was approved for the treatment of patients with locally advanced or metastatic UC who have disease progression during or following platinum-containing chemotherapy, based on findings from KEYNOTE-045, which is the first phase 3 trial to show a significant survival benefit for patients with advanced UC in the second-line setting [37]. KEYNOTE-045 is a multicenter, randomized trial that investigated 542 patients with locally advanced or metastatic urothelial carcinoma that progressed on/after platinum-based chemotherapy. The trial randomized patients to pembrolizumab or one of three single-agent chemotherapy regimens (paclitaxel, docetaxel, or vinflunine), chosen by the investigators. The study demonstrated a statistically significant improvement in OS: 10.1 vs 7.3 HR 0.70 [37, 38]. In June 2019, pembrolizumab was approved as first-line treatment for patients with locally advanced or metastatic urothelial carcinoma who are not eligible for cisplatin-containing chemotherapy and whose tumors express PD-L1 or in patients who are not suitable for chemotherapy regardless of PD-L1 status. The FDA approval was based on the

KEYNOTE-052 trial, where 374 patients with UC who were not eligible for cisplatin-based chemotherapy were enrolled and received at least one dose of pembrolizumab (200 mg every 3 weeks). The median ORR was 29% in all patients, while the PD-L1-expression cutoff of 10% was associated with a higher frequency of response to pembrolizumab as demonstrated by the ORR (21% in PD-L1 CPS <10 subgroups vs 47% of PD-L1 CPS ≥10 subgroups) [39, 40]. Recently, pembrolizumab has been approved for the first-line treatment of patients with advanced renal cell carcinoma (RCC) in combination with axitinib. The approval was based on the results of KEYNOTE-426, a randomized, multicenter, open-label trial conducted in 861 patients who had not received systemic therapy for advanced RCC which compared pembrolizumab plus axitinib versus sunitinib [41]. The combination treatment of pembrolizumab/axitinib resulted in a 47% lower risk of death and a 31% lower risk of disease progression than standard treatment (HR 0.53; 95% CI, 0.38–0.74). The study demonstrated a superior median PFS of 15.1 months for the experimental arm (95% CI, 12.6–17.7) as compared to the sunitinib arm (11.1 months, 95% CI, 8.7–12.5). Interestingly, the benefits of pembrolizumab plus axitinib were observed in all subgroups examined, including PD-L1 expression categories. Notably, in a recent update presented at ASCO 2020 by Plimack, pembrolizumab plus axitinib continued to demonstrate better outcomes as compared with sunitinib at a median follow-up of 27 months, considering median PFS 15.4 months vs 11.1 months; HR 0.71; CI 95% 0.6–0.84) and PFS at 24 months (38% vs 27%) [42]. Anti-PD-1 antibody pembrolizumab showed its efficacy also on gastric and gastroesophageal junction adenocarcinoma (GEJA), as demonstrated by KEYNOTE-059. In this phase II, single-arm and multi-cohort trial, pembrolizumab was investigated in patients who progressed after two or more chemotherapy lines as a single agent (Cohort 1) and in naïve patients both in combination with chemotherapy (Cohort 2) and as a single agent (Cohort 3) [43]. The results demonstrated that pembrolizumab is well-tolerated and has promising antitumor activity in pretreated patients. Recently published, the phase III trial KEYNOTE-062 explored the frontline combination of pembrolizumab+cisplatinum/5FU in PD-L1+ and HER2-negative tumors showing that pembrolizumab was non-inferior to chemotherapy [44]. Following the KEYNOTE-180 and KEYNOTE-181 trials, pembrolizumab was approved for the treatment of patients with recurrent locally advanced or metastatic squamous cell carcinoma of the esophagus whose tumors express PD-L1 with disease progression after one or more prior lines of systemic therapy. KEYNOTE-181 enrolled patients with recurrent locally advanced or metastatic esophageal cancer who progressed on or after one prior line of systemic treatment for advanced disease and on or after at least two prior systemic treatments for advanced disease, comparing pembrolizumab with chemotherapy. Median OS was 9.3 months for pembrolizumab (95% CI, 6.6–12.5) vs 6.7 months for chemotherapy-only arm (HR, 0.69; 95% CI, 0.52–0.93) [45]. KEYNOTE-180 showed durable antitumor activity and manageable safety of pembrolizumab in pretreated patients with metastatic esophageal cancer whose disease progressed after two or more lines of therapy. Of note, among the 35 patients with ESCC expressing PD-L1 CPS ≥10, ORR was 20%, even if the antitumor activity was observed regardless of PD-L1 status [46]. Finally, data from KEYNOTE-590 which is evaluating pembrolizumab plus chemotherapy as first-line therapy for patients with locally advanced or metastatic esophageal carcinoma are still warranted. Preliminary results presented at the ESMO Annual Meeting 2020 showed an improvement in OS and PFS with pembrolizumab in combination with chemotherapy [47]. Among gastrointestinal tumors, pembrolizumab is also indicated for the treatment of patients with hepatocellular carcinoma (HCC) who have been previously treated with sorafenib. This indication is based on tumor response rate and durability of response demonstrated in KEYNOTE-224, a phase II trial in patients with HCC who had disease progression on or after sorafenib or were intolerant to sorafenib [48]. Pembrolizumab was also the first ICI to receive agnostic FDA approval. In May 2017, the FDA approved pembrolizumab for the treatment of adult and pediatric patients with unresectable MSI-H or dMMR solid tumors, regardless of primary tumor or histology. The FDA's approval was based on data from 149 patients with MSI-H or dMMR cancer who were enrolled in five clinical trials (KEYNOTE 12, 164, 158, and 28) [49–51]. Of a total of 149 patients across 15 tumor types, 47 had dMMR, 60 had MSI-H, and 42 had both. The patients were treated with pembrolizumab every 2 or every 3 weeks. The ORR was 39.6% with a total of 11 complete responses and 48 partial responses. The ORR was similar irrespective of histology. More recently, in June 2020, pembrolizumab was approved by the FDA for the treatment of adult and pediatric patients with unresectable or metastatic solid tumors with tissue tumor mutational burden–high (TMB-H; $\geq$10 mutations/megabase), who progressed after prior therapy and have no alternative treatment options. TMB is the number of somatic gene mutations of a tumor. It is suggested that these tumor mutations are associated with the expression of neoantigens. Hence, tumors with a high TMB may be more likely to respond to ICI therapies. In KEYNOTE-158, 102 patients had TMB-H tumors, and they showed ORR of 29% (95% CI: 21.39). Marabelle et al. further explored the relationship between antitumor activity and TMB in a prospective analysis of the phase 2 KEYNOTE-158 study, reporting an ORR of 28.3% for TMB-high (24.8% (16.9–34.1) non–MSI-H) and 6.5% (4.7–8.7) for TMB-low. Median OS for TMB-high and low was 11.1 mo (8.1–16.1) and 13.3 mo (11.5–14.8), respectively; 12-month rates were 48.0% and 52.9%. TMB-high was associated with higher ORR in pts. with select advanced solid tumors treated with pembrolizumab monotherapy [51].

Moreover, in June 2020, pembrolizumab was approved for first-line treatment of patients with unresectable or metastatic MSI-H or dMMR colorectal cancer. Approval was based on KEYNOTE-177, which compared pembrolizumab with mFOLFOX6/FOLFIRI $\pm$ bevacizumab or cetuximab, demonstrating a significant improvement in PFS (16.5 months vs 8.2 months). The subgroup analysis showed a promising RR of 50.0% with first-line pembrolizumab and 31.9% in pretreated patients [52]. Concerning gynecological cancers, pembrolizumab is indicated for the treatment of recurrent or metastatic cervical cancer with PD-L1 $\geq$ 1, based on the results from a single cohort of the KEYNOTE-158 study which demonstrated a durable antitumor activity and manageable safety in this population of patients. Indeed, 98 patients affected by recurrent or metastatic cervical cancer were included in a single cohort (Cohort E). The 12 responses occurred in patients with PD-L1–positive tumors, for an ORR of 14.6%. Furthermore, pembrolizumab plus lenvatinib is approved for the treatment of advanced endometrial carcinoma, not MSI-H or dMMR, in patients who have progressed after prior systemic therapy, yet not candidates for surgery or radiation. KEYNOTE-146 enrolled 108 patients with metastatic endometrial carcinoma who progressed after treatment. ORR was 38.3% (95% CI 28.5–48.9%) with 10 complete responses. About HNSCC, the introduction of monoclonal antibodies in the treatment landscape was a turning point for patients that had a 50% recurrence rate, despite aggressive multimodality treatment (surgery, radiotherapy, chemotherapy, EGFR inhibitors) [53]. Pembrolizumab was initially approved as a single agent for the treatment of patients with recurrent or metastatic HNSCC with disease progression on or after platinum-containing chemotherapy, following the KEYNOTE-012. The study demonstrated an ORR of 18% (8/45 patients) and was 25% (4/16 patients) in HPV-positive patients and 14% (4/29 patients) in HPV-negative patients [54]. Afterward, pembrolizumab was approved for the first-line treatment of patients with metastatic or with unresectable, recurrent HNSCC whose tumors express PD-L1 $\geq$ 1 as a single agent and in combination with platinum and fluorouracil. KEYNOTE-048 enrolled patients stratified by tumor PD-L1 expression $\geq$50% or < 50%, HPV status, and ECOG PS. Patients were stratified to receive pembrolizumab ($n = 301$), pembrolizumab with platinum and 5-FU ($n = 281$), or cetuximab with platinum and 5-FU ($n = 300$). The study demonstrated a statistically significant improvement in OS for the subgroup of patients with PD-L1 CPS $\geq$1 randomized to pembrolizumab monotherapy [55].

Nivolumab

Nivolumab is a completely human immunoglobulin G4 monoclonal antibody which targets PD-1.

Clinical indications of nivolumab include the treatment of various solid tumors and hematological cancers: melanoma, NSCLC, SCLC, RCC, HNSCC, UC, MSI-H, or dMMR mCRC, HCC, and esophageal squamous cell carcinoma.

However, nivolumab is currently approved for unresectable or metastatic melanoma as a single agent or in combination with ipilimumab and in the adjuvant setting for patients with lymph node involvement or metastatic disease who have undergone complete resection. CheckMate 037, which compared nivolumab with chemotherapy, led to FDA approval as a second-line or later-line treatment in patients with advanced melanoma. Indeed, ORR was superior in the IO arm, with 38/120 pts in the nivolumab arm (31.7%) vs 5/47 pts (10.6%) in the chemotherapy arm [56]. Thereupon, CheckMate 066 aimed to assess the efficacy and safety of nivolumab in pts with previously untreated melanoma without a *BRAF* mutation. The trial demonstrated the superiority of nivolumab over standard chemotherapy treatment, with a PFS of 5.1 mo. vs 2.2 mo. (95% CI, 2.1–2.4) [57]. Moreover, to achieve a more durable and long-lasting treatment response, combinations of ICIs have been explored in various settings. CheckMate 067 compared the efficacy and safety of single-agent nivolumab and the combination regimen (nivolumab plus ipilimumab) compared to ipilimumab. The study demonstrated a significant improvement in objective responses, progression-free survival, and overall survival with the nivolumab plus ipilimumab combination. PFS was significantly longer in the combination therapy with an HR of 0.42 (95% CI 0.35–0.51) [58]. These results were confirmed by the CheckMate 067 trial. Based on the findings of CheckMate 238, the indication of nivolumab was extended to the adjuvant setting of melanoma. This randomized trial demonstrated the superiority of nivolumab compared with ipilimumab in terms of RFS with an HR of 0.65 (97% CI, 0.51–0.83) [59].

Moreover, with a reference to NSCLC, nivolumab was firstly investigated in CheckMate 017, an open-label phase III trial that enrolled patients with metastatic squamous NSCLC who had experienced disease progression during or after platinum-based chemotherapy, regardless of PD-L1 status. The trial demonstrated a statistically significant improvement in OS for patients randomized to nivolumab as compared with docetaxel (9.2 mo. in the nivolumab group vs 6 mo. in the docetaxel group) [60]. Furthermore, the CheckMate 057 trial enrolled 582 patients, evaluating the efficacy of nivolumab as compared with docetaxel. The trial demonstrated the superiority of nivolumab with significantly longer OS (12.2 vs 9.4 mo.), representing a 27% lower risk of death with nivolumab. The benefit of nivolumab was observed in the overall population, but the greatness of benefit across all the efficacy endpoints appeared to be greater among patients whose tumors expressed PD-L1 than among PD-L1 negative. Both aforementioned studies met their primary endpoints of demonstrating improved overall survival compared with docetaxel, and they represented a milestone for the treatment of patients with NSCLC whose disease had progressed to prior chemotherapy, which changed the therapeutic approach in this population of patients. Combinations of ICIs have been explored also in NSCLC, aiming to improve the duration of response to treatments; thus, in May 2020, nivolumab was approved as first-line treatment in adult patients with metastatic non–small cell lung cancer expressing PD-L1 in combination with ipilimumab, thanks to the findings from the CheckMate 227. Median OS was 17.1 months vs 14.9 months, HR 0.79 [61]. Notably, this trial was the first to examine the clinical utility of TMB as a predictive biomarker of the response to immunotherapy in the first-line setting of advanced NSCLC. However, as reported by different authors, TMB seemed to not be ready for standard clinical practice [47]. Moreover, the combination of nivolumab+ipilimumab was investigated in the CheckMate 9LA, where naïve NSCLC pts. were treated with nivolumab and ipilimumab followed by a subsequent limited course of chemotherapy. Median OS was 14.1 vs 10.7 mo. with a significant HR for death of 0.69 in favor of the combination arm. The 1-year OS rates were 63% and 47%, respectively. Subgroup analysis indicated that the combination regimen prolonged the OS regardless of the histology. Referring to urological malignancies, the historical treatment of metastatic renal cell carcinoma, based on the use of antiangiogenic agents, was revolutionized by nivolumab, as in 2015 nivolumab was approved by the FDA for the treatment of mRCC in second-line setting. The study which led to this approval was CheckMate 025, which compared nivolumab with everolimus demonstrating a statistically significant improvement in

OS for patients randomized to nivolumab as compared with everolimus. mOS was 25.0 months with nivolumab vs 19.6 months with everolimus (HR 0.73 95% CI, 0.57–0.93). The median PFS was 4.6 months with nivolumab and 4.4 months with everolimus (HR 0.88; 95% CI, 0.75–1.03) [62].

However, sunitinib, a vascular endothelial growth factor receptor (VEGFR) TKI, was a standard of care for first-line treatment of advanced renal-cell carcinoma for decades, until 2018 when the results of CheckMate 214 were published. Indeed, Motzer et al. investigated the combination of nivolumab and ipilimumab as first-line treatment for patients with intermediate or poor risk, with advanced RCC. This open-label trial demonstrated a significant superiority in OS as well as ORR of the combination as compared with sunitinib. Notably, a longer OS and a higher ORR were observed with the combination of ICIs, especially among intermediate- and poor-risk patients across tumor PD-L1 expression levels, although the magnitude of benefit was higher in the population with 1% or greater PD-L1 expression. Additionally, ICIs targeting the PD-1/PD-L1 pathway have shown their efficacy also in gastrointestinal cancers. In fact, in June 2020, nivolumab was approved for the treatment of patients with unresectable advanced, recurrent, or metastatic ESCC after prior fluoropyrimidine- and platinum-based chemotherapy based on findings from ATTRACTION-3, a multicenter, randomized, active-controlled, open-label trial. Median OS was 10.9 months vs 8.4 months with a 23% reduction in risk of death (HR 0.77 95% CI 0.62–0.96). However, an overall HR of 1.08 (95%, CI 0.87–1.34) suggested no meaningful difference in PFS between nivolumab and the chemotherapy arm [63].

Furthermore, nivolumab as a single agent or in combination with ipilimumab is indicated as second-line treatment for MSI-H or dMMR mCRC progressed following treatment with a fluoropyrimidine, oxaliplatin, and irinotecan. Metastatic dMMR/MSI-H mCRC has a poor prognosis after the failure of the initial treatment with standard chemotherapy. Nonetheless, due to high levels of tumor neoantigens, tumor-infiltrating lymphocytes, and checkpoint regulators, these tumors respond to PD-1 blockade. For this reason, nivolumab demonstrated durable responses, disease control, and long-term survival in pretreated patients with dMMR/MSI-H mCRC, representing a new treatment option for these patients. CheckMate 142 evaluated nivolumab monotherapy in a cohort of 75 patients, 53 of which (71.6%) had MSI-H tumors, and 14 (18.9%) did not have MSI-H tumors [64].

Anti-PD-L1 Agents

Atezolizumab

Atezolizumab is a monoclonal antibody that binds to PD-L1 and blocks its interaction with PD-1. It was firstly approved by the FDA in 2016 for the treatment of platinum-resistant metastatic NSCLC. In this setting, atezolizumab approval was based on the clinical benefit shown in the phase III OAK trial, consistent with the data from the phase II POPLAR study [65]. In these studies, atezolizumab significantly prolonged OS as compared to docetaxel, regardless of PD-L1 status. Indeed, in the ITT population, OS was greater with atezolizumab vs docetaxel (HR 0.73 95% CI 0.62–0.87), and the benefit was seen regardless of PD-L1 [66]. Consequently, further trials were conducted to evaluate atezolizumab in treatment-naïve NSCLC patients. IMpower130 investigated the efficacy and safety of atezolizumab plus chemotherapy vs chemotherapy alone. Median OS was 18.6 months in the atezolizumab group vs 13.9 months in the chemotherapy group and a median PFS of 7.0 months vs 5.5 months [67]. Based on these results, atezolizumab was approved in combination with bevacizumab, paclitaxel, and carboplatin, for the first-line treatment of adult patients with metastatic non-squamous NSCLC with no EGFR or ALK genomic tumor aberrations [68]. Considering that the efficacy of atezolizumab may be empowered by the blockade of VEGFR–mediated immuno-suppression, the combo of atezolizumab plus bevacizumab was investigated in the IMpower150, an open-label, phase 3 study in treatment-naïve patients. The patients were randomized to receive atezolizumab plus carboplatin plus paclitaxel, bevacizumab plus carboplatin plus paclitaxel, or atezolizumab plus bevacizumab, carboplatin, and paclitaxel every 3 weeks for four or six cycles, followed by maintenance therapy with atezolizumab, bevacizumab, or both. The study demonstrated that the addition of atezolizumab to bevacizumab plus chemotherapy for metastatic NSCLC resulted in a significant improvement in PFS and OS, regardless of PD-L1 expression including in the PD-L1-negative subgroup (7.1 months vs. 6.9 months HR 0.77 95% CI, 0.61–0.99) and the PD-L1–low subgroup (8.3 months vs. 6.6 months HR 0.56 95% CI, 0.41–0.77). Recently, atezolizumab was approved for the first-line treatment of patients with metastatic NSCLC whose tumors have a PD-L1 expression ≥50% [69]. The efficacy of atezolizumab in the abovementioned setting was evaluated in IMpower110, a multicenter, international, randomized, open-label trial that assigned patients to atezolizumab or platinum-based chemotherapy. The trial demonstrated a statistically significant improvement in OS for patients with high PD-L1 expression (20.2 months vs 13.1 months HR 0.59; 95% CI: 0.40, 0.89). PFS showed an HR of 0.63 (95% CI: 0.45, 0.88), with a median PFS of 8.1 months (95% CI: 6.8, 11.0) in the atezolizumab arm and 5 months (95% CI: 4.2, 5.7) in the platinum-based chemotherapy arm. ORR was 38% in the atezolizumab arm and 29% in the platinum-based chemotherapy arm.

Moreover, atezolizumab showed a crucial role in SCLC, a disease with a poor prognosis, proving itself as a milestone for the management of SCLC patients. The efficacy of atezolizumab plus carboplatin and etoposide was investigated in IMpower133, a multicenter, double-blind, placebo-controlled trial that compared atezolizumab plus carboplatin and etoposide with placebo plus the standard-of-care [70]. The study demonstrated a significant statistical improvement for the atezolizumab arm both in terms of PFS (5.2 vs 4.3 months, HR = 0.77) and OS (12.3 months vs 10.3 months) with HR = 0.70. However, atezolizumab could promote sustained responses in urothelial carcinoma. Indeed, in May 2016, FDA approved atezolizumab for the treatment of patients with locally advanced or metastatic urothelial carcinoma whose disease progressed during or following platinum-containing chemotherapy or within 12 months of neoadjuvant or adjuvant treatment with platinum-containing chemotherapy. The IMvigor 210 trial tested the efficacy of atezolizumab in two cohorts of patients: patients who progressed during or following a prior platinum-based chemotherapy regimen, whereas the other cohort included treatment-naïve patients with advanced urothelial carcinoma who were ineligible for cisplatin-containing chemotherapy. The study showed an ORR of 23%. Of note, responses occurred across all PD-L1 subgroups. The median PFS was 2.7 months and the median OS was 15.9 months. Considering the results, atezolizumab was approved for locally advanced or metastatic urothelial carcinoma not eligible for cisplatin and whose tumors express PD-L1. Immunotherapies targeting the PD-L1–PD-1 pathway in combination with anti-VEGF have been currently evaluated in hepatocellular carcinoma (HCC). Additionally, based on the IMbrave150 study, atezolizumab is indicated in combination with bevacizumab for treatment-naïve patients with unresectable or metastatic HCC. Thus, 501 patients with unresectable or metastatic HCC received atezolizumab plus bevacizumab or sorafenib. The study met the two co-primary endpoints with a median OS that had not been reached at the time of the analysis for atezolizumab plus bevacizumab compared to 13.2 months for patients randomized to sorafenib. Of note, HR for OS was 0.58 (95% CI 0.42, 0.79), median PFS was significantly increased (6.8 vs 4.3 months, HR 0.59, 95% CI 0.47–0.76) [71]. Further, atezolizumab was demonstrated to have a manageable safety profile and clinical activity in patients with other solid tumors, including triple-negative breast cancer (TNBC). Moreover, chemotherapy might empower tumor-antigen release and antitumor responses to ICIs. In the light of this consideration, Impassion130, a phase 3 multicenter, randomized trial, included 902 unresectable or metastatic treatment-naïve TNBC and was randomly assigned to receive atezolizumab or placebo plus nab-paclitaxel. The study demonstrated a significantly longer PFS in the atezolizumab group both in the ITT and in the patients with positive PDL-1 [72]. Median PFS was 7.2 months vs. 5.5 months in the ITT population (HR 0.80, 0.69–0.92) and 7.5 months vs 5.0 months in the PDL-1 positive subgroup (HR 0.62). The median OS was 10 months longer than the placebo subgroup (25.0 months vs 15.5 months; HR 0.62). Finally, the objective response rate was higher with the combination compared to chemotherapy alone for all patients (56% vs 46%) and those with PD-L1–positive tumors (59% vs 43%). Therefore, atezolizumab plus paclitaxel protein-bound is indicated for the treatment of unresectable or metastatic PD-L1 -positive TNBC.

Durvalumab

Durvalumab is a PD-L1 blocking antibody that has several applications in different tumors such as urothelial carcinoma, NSCLC, extensive-stage SCLC (ES-SCLC). Firstly, in 2017, the FDA has granted accelerated approval to durvalumab for the treatment of patients with locally advanced or metastatic urothelial cancer who have disease progression during or after platinum-containing chemotherapy or whose disease has progressed within 12 months or after surgery. The efficacy of durvalumab was evaluated in the urothelial carcinoma cohort of Study 1108, a multicenter, multi-cohort, open-label clinical trial phase I/II [73]. A total of 182 patients with locally advanced or metastatic urothelial carcinoma progressed after treatment were enrolled and received durvalumab every 2 weeks up to 12 months. In the study, durvalumab has demonstrated an ORR of 17.0% (95% CI: 11.9–23.3) in all patients, regardless of PD-L1 status, and 26.3% (95% CI: 17.8–36.4) in patients with high-expression PD-L1 tumors. In addition, approximately 14.3% ($n = 26$) and 2.7% ($n = 5$) of all patients had a partial response and a complete response, respectively. The median PFS and OS were 1.5 months (95% CI 1.4–1.9 months) and 18.2 months (95% CI 8.1 months to NE), respectively. At 1 year, the OS rate was 55% (95% CI, 44–65%).

As abovementioned, immunotherapy has completely changed the treatment landscape of thoracic malignancies. Notably, durvalumab was the first ICI to demonstrate a clinical benefit after chemoradiotherapy treatment in stage III NSCLC. The efficacy of durvalumab was evaluated in the PACIFIC study, a multicenter, randomized, double-blind, placebo-controlled study in patients with unresectable stage III NSCLC who completed at least two cycles of concurrent platinum-based chemotherapy and definitive radiation within 42 days before the initiation of the study drug [74]. The patients were randomized 2:1 to receive durvalumab or placebo every 2 weeks for up to 12 months. Therefore, the median PFS from randomization was 16.8 months (95% CI, 13.0–18.1) with durvalumab vs 5.6 months (95% CI, 4.6–7.8) with placebo (HR 0.52; 95% CI, 0.42–0.65). OS rates at 12, 24, and 36 months were in favor of durvalumab (83.1% vs 74.6%, 66.3% vs 55.3%, and 57.0% vs 43.5%, respectively). Noteworthy, the stratified HR for risk of death and progression of disease was 0.68 (95% CI, 0.53–0.87) and 0.52, respectively. The median time to death or distant metastasis was longer with durvalumab than with placebo (23.2 months vs. 14.6 months). Additional subgroup analyses were conducted, and the safety profile of durvalumab in the PD-L1 TC subgroup ≥1% was consistent with the ITT population, as was the subgroup with PD-L1 TC <1%. Of note, an updated 4-year analysis from PACIFIC, recently presented at ESMO congress 2020, confirmed the significant benefit in OS and PFS reported at the time of the primary analyses with a durable PFS and sustained OS benefit [75].

Moreover, in 2020, durvalumab was approved as a first-line treatment for adult patients with (ES-SCLC in combination with the standard-of-care (platinum-etoposide). Indeed, the CASPIAN study, an international, randomized, and open-label multicenter trial, evaluated the impact of adding durvalumab to chemotherapy [76]. The 805 patients enrolled were equally assigned to three arms: durvalumab plus platinum-etoposide, durvalumab plus tremelimumab plus platinum-etoposide, or platinum-etoposide alone. Of note, durvalumab plus chemotherapy demonstrated a statistically significant and clinically meaningful improvement in OS vs platinum-etoposide alone (13 months (95% CI 11.5–14.8) vs 10.3 months (9.3–11.2) with an HR of 0.73 (95% CI 0.59–0.91). Noteworthy, the updated data presented at the ASCO 2020 Virtual Congress continued to confirm the benefit of the combination therapy in comparison with chemotherapy alone with a median OS of 12.9 months (95% CI 11.3–14.7) in the durvalumab plus platinum-etoposide arm vs 10.5 months (CI 95%, 9.3–11.2) in the arm treated with chemotherapy (HR 0.75; 95% CI,

0.62–0.91). Contrarywise, durvalumab, and tremelimumab with the chemotherapy arm were not superior to chemotherapy alone in terms of survival (median OS was 10.4 months vs 10.5 months in the chemo arm (HR 0.82; 95% CI 0.68–1.00)). Due to these results, the FDA, and afterward EMA, approved durvalumab in combination with chemotherapy as first-line therapy for patients with ES-SCLC.

Avelumab

Avelumab is a human IgG1 monoclonal antibody directed against the death receptor ligand PD-L1. Avelumab is indicated in combination with axitinib for the first-line treatment of patients affected by metastatic RCC and metastatic urothelial carcinoma. The last approval was based on the results from the phase III JAVELIN Bladder 100 study investigating first-line maintenance treatment with avelumab plus best supportive care (BSC) vs BSC alone in patients with locally advanced or metastatic urothelial carcinoma who have not progressed to first-line platinum-containing chemotherapy. A total of 700 patients were randomly assigned to receive avelumab plus BSC or BSC alone. This study has demonstrated a significant 7.1-month improvement in median OS with avelumab plus BSC versus BSC alone: 21.4 months (95% CI: 18.9–26.1) vs 14.3 months (95% CI: 12.9–17.9). This statistically significant improvement in OS represents a 31% reduction in the risk of death in the overall population (HR 0.69; 95% CI: 0.56–0.86). In PD-L1+ patients ($n = 358$, 51%), the risk of death was reduced by 44% in the avelumab arm compared to the control arm (HR 0.56; 95% CI: 0.40–0.79). Moreover, in 2019, the FDA approved avelumab in combination with axitinib for the first-line treatment of patients with metastatic RCC. The approval was based on positive results from the phase III JAVELIN Renal 101 study, a randomized, multicenter, open-label, which involved 886 patients with untreated advanced RCC regardless of tumor PD-L1 expression [62]. Patients were randomized to one of the following treatment arms: avelumab in combination with axitinib or sunitinib. The combination of avelumab and axitinib significantly improved median PFS compared to sunitinib by more than 5 months (HR: 0.69; 95% CI: 0.56–0.84); median PFS for avelumab in combination with axitinib by 13.8 months [95% CI: 11.1- NE], and sunitinib by 8.4 months [95% CI: 6.9–11.1]. The ORR was doubled in the ITT population with avelumab in combination with axitinib compared to sunitinib (51.4% (95% CI: 46.6–56.1) vs 25.7% (95% CI: 21.7–30.0)).

Anti-CTLA4 Agents

Ipilimumab

Ipilimumab is a full human cytotoxic T-lymphocyte antigen 4 (CTLA-4)-blocking antibody. To date, its indications include the treatment of metastatic melanoma; intermediate or poor-risk, previously untreated metastatic renal cell carcinoma, in combination with nivolumab; treatment of adult and pediatric patients 12 years of age and older with (MSI-H) or mismatch repair-deficient (dMMR) metastatic colorectal cancer that has progressed following treatment with a fluoropyrimidine, oxaliplatin, and irinotecan, in combination with nivolumab; and treatment of patients with hepatocellular carcinoma who have been previously treated with sorafenib, in combination with nivolumab. The introduction of checkpoint inhibitor drugs has represented a breakthrough in the treatment of melanoma [77]. Recently, nivolumab and pembrolizumab have been introduced in the treatment landscape of melanoma, obtaining refundability in 2016 for the treatment of unresectable stages IV or III, after CheckMate 037 and CheckMate 066. Subsequently, several clinical trials were conducted on the combination of ipilimumab and nivolumab. The CheckMate 067 is a double-blind, randomized phase III study comparing the combination of nivolumab + ipilimumab to monotherapy with nivolumab vs ipilimumab in unresectable melanoma treatment-naïve patients. At a minimum follow-up of 60 months, the combination treatment was superior in terms of PFS (HR 0.42, 95% CI 0.35–0.51), OS (HR 0.63, 95% CI 0.42–0.64), and RR (58% vs 19%, 95% CI 53–64, 15–24, respectively) vs ipilimumab. However, toxicities were higher in the combination arm (59% versus 23% and 28% for nivolumab and ipilimumab, respectively) [58]. Currently, the combination has obtained a positive opinion from the EMA, but it is not refundable among all European countries. However, ipilimumab has a role also in the adjuvant treatment of melanoma. In October 2015, the FDA approved ipilimumab in the adjuvant setting for melanoma patients with regional lymph node involvement of >1 mm after complete resection. The approval was granted after the published results of the CA184–029 study [78]. In this randomized, double-blind, placebo-controlled trial, patients with resected stage III A, B, and C cutaneous melanoma were randomized to receive after standard adjuvant treatment, ipilimumab every 12 weeks for 3 years as maintenance therapy, or placebo. The authors reported a significantly improved RFS in the ipilimumab arm compared to the placebo. The median RFS of 27.6 months (95% CI:19.3–37.2) compared to 17.1 months (95% CI:13.6–21.6), respectively (HR = 0.76; 95% CI: 0.64–0.89). Estimated five-OS rate of 65.4% (95% CI: 60.8–69.6) for ipilimumab vs 54.4% (95% CI: 49.7–58.9) for placebo. Additionally, the analysis confirmed the safety profile, yet the immune-related adverse events were more frequent with ipilimumab than with placebo.

Ipilimumab was investigated also in combination with nivolumab, as abovementioned. Notably, the combination of anti-PD-1 and anti-CTLA-4 led recently to the EMA approval as a first-line treatment strategy in advanced RCC treatment-naïve patients. CheckMate 214 study included intermediate and poor-risk patients according to the International Metastatic RCC Criteria Consortium Database (IMDC). Patients were randomized to nivolumab plus ipilimumab every 3 weeks for four cycles, followed by maintenance with nivolumab or to sunitinib. The trial study showed important clinical responses, median PFS, and longer OS than in the sunitinib arm, still with a manageable safety profile. The immunotherapy combination was also explored in metastatic CRC with dMMR and in patients with MSI-H [79]. CheckMate 142, a multicenter, non-randomized, open-label clinical trial, enrolled 82 patients with dMMR or MSI-H mCRC after disease progression. All patients received ipilimumab and nivolumab every 3 weeks for four cycles, followed by nivolumab monotherapy every 2 weeks, achieving complete responses in 9% and 18%, and DCR was 84% and 78%, respectively. At a follow-up time of 15 months, 75% of patients were progression-free, and 84% were alive. Moreover, the results for treatment-naïve patients with MSI-H mCRC showed an ORR of 60% and up to 7% of the ITT displayed a complete response. The 12-month PFS and OS rates were 77% and 83%, respectively. These data further support the potential use of the immunotherapy combination in the first line in this particular population. The novel and effective combination of ICIs has shown its efficacy also in unresectable malignant pleural mesothelioma (MPM). Indeed, the phase 3 CheckMate 743, an open-label, multicenter, randomized study, evaluated nivolumab plus ipilimumab vs standard chemotherapy in patients with MPM. The combo demonstrated superior OS compared to standard-of-care platinum-based chemotherapy (HR: 0.74 95% CI: 0.61–0.89), with a median OS of 18.1 months compared to 14.1 months, respectively. These results were observed after 22.1 months of minimum follow-up. At 2 years, 41% of patients treated with the combo were alive and 27% with chemotherapy.

References

1. Twomey JD, Zhang B. Cancer immunotherapy update: FDA-approved checkpoint inhibitors and companion diagnostics. AAPS J. 2021;23(2):39. https://doi.org/10.1208/s12248-021-00574-0.
2. Russo A, et al. The tumor-agnostic treatment for patients with solid tumors: a position paper on behalf of the AIOM- SIAPEC/IAP-SIBioC-SIF Italian Scientific Societies. Crit Rev Oncol Hematol. 2021;165:103436. https://doi.org/10.1016/j.critrevonc.2021.103436.
3. Incorvaia L, et al. Baseline plasma levels of soluble PD-1, PD-L1, and BTN3A1 predict response to nivolumab treatment in patients with metastatic renal cell carcinoma: a step toward a biomarker for therapeutic decisions. Oncoimmunology. 2020;9(1):1832348. https://doi.org/10.1080/2162402X.2020.1832348.
4. Badalamenti G, et al. Role of tumor-infiltrating lymphocytes in patients with solid tumors: can a drop dig a stone? Cell Immunol. 2019;343:103753. https://doi.org/10.1016/j.cellimm.2018.01.013.
5. Banstola A, Jeong J-H, Yook S. Immunoadjuvants for cancer immunotherapy: a review of recent developments. Acta Biomater. 2020;114:16–30. https://doi.org/10.1016/j.actbio.2020.07.063.
6. Russo A, et al. The molecular profiling of solid tumors by liquid biopsy: a position paper of the AIOM-SIAPEC-IAP-SIBioC-SIC-SIF Italian Scientific Societies. ESMO Open. 2021;6(3):100164. https://doi.org/10.1016/j.esmoop.2021.100164.
7. Incorvaia L, et al. Programmed death ligand 1 (PD-L1) as a predictive biomarker for pembrolizumab therapy in patients with advanced non-small-cell lung cancer (NSCLC). Adv Ther. 2019; https://doi.org/10.1007/s12325-019-01057-7.
8. Marcus L, Lemery SJ, Keegan P, Pazdur R. FDA approval summary: pembrolizumab for the treatment of microsatellite instability-high solid tumors'. Clin Cancer Res. 2019;25(13):3753–8. https://doi.org/10.1158/1078-0432.CCR-18-4070.
9. Galvano A, et al. The prognostic impact of tumor mutational burden (TMB) in the first-line management of advanced non-oncogene addicted non-small-cell lung cancer (NSCLC): a systematic review and meta-analysis of randomized controlled trials. ESMO Open. 2021;6(3) https://doi.org/10.1016/j.esmoop.2021.100124.

10. Emancipator K. Keytruda and PD-L1: a real-world example of co-development of a drug with a predictive biomarker. AAPS J. 2020;23(1):5. https://doi.org/10.1208/s12248-020-00525-1.
11. Novo G, et al. Arterial stiffness: effects of anticancer drugs used for breast cancer women. Front Physiol. 2021;12:661464. https://doi.org/10.3389/fphys.2021.661464.
12. Lee KA, Nathan P. Cutaneous melanoma – a review of systemic therapies. Acta Derm Venereol. 2020;100(11):adv00141. https://doi.org/10.2340/00015555-3496.
13. Ribas A, et al. Pembrolizumab versus investigator-choice chemotherapy for ipilimumab-refractory melanoma (KEYNOTE-002): a randomised, controlled, phase 2 trial. Lancet Oncol. 2015;16(8):908–18. https://doi.org/10.1016/S1470-2045(15)00083-2.
14. Hamid O, et al. Five-year survival outcomes for patients with advanced melanoma treated with pembrolizumab in KEYNOTE-001. Ann Oncol Off J Eur Soc Med Oncol. 2019;30(4):582–8. https://doi.org/10.1093/annonc/mdz011.
15. Gristina V, La Mantia M, Iacono F, Galvano A, Russo A, Bazan V. The emerging therapeutic landscape of ALK inhibitors in non-small cell lung cancer. Pharmaceuticals (Basel). 2020;13(12) https://doi.org/10.3390/ph13120474.
16. Gristina V, et al. Non-small cell lung cancer harboring concurrent EGFR genomic alterations: a systematic review and critical appraisal of the double dilemma. J Mol Pathol. 2021;2(2):173–96. https://doi.org/10.3390/jmp2020016.
17. Pepe F, et al. Tumor mutational burden on cytological samples: a pilot study. Cancer Cytopathol. 2020; https://doi.org/10.1002/cncy.22400.
18. Robert C, et al. Pembrolizumab versus ipilimumab in advanced melanoma (KEYNOTE-006): post-hoc 5-year results from an open-label, multicentre, randomised, controlled, phase 3 study. Lancet Oncol. 2019;20(9):1239–51. https://doi.org/10.1016/S1470-2045(19)30388-2.
19. Gristina V, et al. Is there any room for PD-1 inhibitors in combination with platinum-based chemotherapy as frontline treatment of extensive-stage small cell lung cancer? A systematic review and meta-analysis with indirect comparisons among subgroups and landmark survival analyses. Ther Adv Med Oncol. 2021;13:17588359211018018. https://doi.org/10.1177/17588359211018018.
20. Eggermont AMM, et al. Adjuvant pembrolizumab versus placebo in resected stage III melanoma (EORTC 1325-MG/KEYNOTE-054): distant metastasis-free survival results from a double-blind, randomised, controlled, phase 3 trial. Lancet Oncol. 2021;22(5):643–54. https://doi.org/10.1016/S1470-2045(21)00065-6.
21. Incorvaia L, et al. BRCA1/2 pathogenic variants in triple-negative versus luminal-like breast cancers: genotype-phenotype correlation in a cohort of 531 patient. Ther Adv Med Oncol. 2020;12:1758835920975326. https://doi.org/10.1177/1758835920975326.
22. Passiglia F, et al. Is there any place for PD-1/CTLA-4 inhibitors combination in the first-line treatment of advanced NSCLC?-a trial-level meta-analysis in PD-L1 selected subgroups. Transl Lung Cancer Res. 2021;10(7):3106–19. https://doi.org/10.21037/tlcr-21-52.
23. Memon H, Patel BM. Immune checkpoint inhibitors in non-small cell lung cancer: a bird's eye view. Life Sci. 2019;233:116713. https://doi.org/10.1016/j.lfs.2019.116713.
24. Herbst RS, et al. Pembrolizumab versus docetaxel for previously treated, PD-L1-positive, advanced non-small-cell lung cancer (KEYNOTE-010): a randomised controlled trial. Lancet. 2016; https://doi.org/10.1016/S0140-6736(15)01281-7.
25. Reck M, et al. Nivolumab (NIVO) + ipilimumab (IPI) + 2 cycles of platinum-doublet chemotherapy (chemo) vs 4 cycles chemo as first-line (1L) treatment (tx) for stage IV/recurrent non-small cell lung cancer (NSCLC): CheckMate 9LA. J Clin Oncol. 2020; https://doi.org/10.1200/jco.2020.38.15_suppl.9501.
26. Russo A, et al. Neutrophil-to-lymphocyte ratio (NLR), platelet-to-lymphocyte ratio (PLR), and outcomes with nivolumab in pretreated non-small cell lung cancer (NSCLC): a large retrospective multicenter study. Adv Ther. 2020;37(3):1145–55. https://doi.org/10.1007/s12325-020-01229-w.
27. Pisapia P, et al. A narrative review on the implementation of liquid biopsy as a diagnostic tool in thoracic tumors during the COVID-19 pandemic. Mediastinum. 2021;5. [Online]. Available: https://med.amegroups.com/article/view/6433

28. Mok TSK, et al. Pembrolizumab versus chemotherapy for previously untreated, PD-L1-expressing, locally advanced or metastatic non-small-cell lung cancer (KEYNOTE-042): a randomised, open-label, controlled, phase 3 trial. Lancet. 2019; https://doi.org/10.1016/S0140-6736(18)32409-7.

29. Gandhi L, et al. KEYNOTE 189 (adeno): pembrolizumab plus chemotherapy (carbo/pemetrexed) in metastatic non–small-cell lung cancer (adeno). N Engl J Med. 2018; https://doi.org/10.1056/NEJMoa1801005.

30. Gadgeel S, et al. Updated analysis from KEYNOTE-189: pembrolizumab or placebo plus pemetrexed and platinum for previously untreated metastatic nonsquamous non-small-cell lung cancer. J Clin Oncol Off J Am Soc Clin Oncol. 2020;38(14):1505–17. https://doi.org/10.1200/JCO.19.03136.

31. Brunetti O, Derakhshani A, Baradaran B, Galvano A, Russo A, Silvestris N. COVID-19 infection in cancer patients: how can oncologists deal with these patients? Front Oncol. 2020;10:734. https://doi.org/10.3389/fonc.2020.00734.

32. Paz-Ares LG, et al. PARAMOUNT: final overall survival results of the phase III study of maintenance pemetrexed versus placebo immediately after induction treatment with pemetrexed plus cisplatin for advanced nonsquamous non-small-cell lung cancer. J Clin Oncol. 2013; https://doi.org/10.1200/JCO.2012.47.1102.

33. H. C. Chung et al., 'Pembrolizumab after two or more lines of previous therapy in patients with recurrent or metastatic SCLC: results from the KEYNOTE-028 and KEYNOTE-158 studies.', J Thorac Oncol Off Publ Int Assoc Study Lung Cancer, vol. 15, no. 4, pp. 618–627, 2020, doi: https://doi.org/10.1016/j.jtho.2019.12.109.

34. Galvano A, et al. Analysis of systemic inflammatory biomarkers in neuroendocrine carcinomas of the lung: prognostic and predictive significance of NLR, LDH, ALI, and LIPI score. Ther Adv Med Oncol. 2020;12:1758835920942378–10.1177/1758835920942378.

35. Ghatalia P, Zibelman M, Geynisman DM, Plimack E. Approved checkpoint inhibitors in bladder cancer: which drug should be used when? Ther Adv Med Oncol. 2018;10:1758835918788310. https://doi.org/10.1177/1758835918788310.

36. Passiglia F, et al. The diagnostic accuracy of circulating tumor DNA for the detection of EGFR-T790M mutation in NSCLC: a systematic review and meta-analysis. Sci Rep. 2018;8(1):13379. https://doi.org/10.1038/s41598-018-30780-4.

37. Fradet Y, et al. Randomized phase III KEYNOTE-045 trial of pembrolizumab versus paclitaxel, docetaxel, or vinflunine in recurrent advanced urothelial cancer: results of >2 years of follow-up. Ann Oncol Off J Eur Soc Med Oncol. 2019;30(6):970–6. https://doi.org/10.1093/annonc/mdz127.

38. Galvano A, et al. Detection of RAS mutations in circulating tumor DNA: a new weapon in an old war against colorectal cancer. A systematic review of literature and meta-analysis. Ther Adv Med Oncol. 2019;11:1758835919874653. https://doi.org/10.1177/1758835919874653.

39. Balar AV, et al. First-line pembrolizumab in cisplatin-ineligible patients with locally advanced and unresectable or metastatic urothelial cancer (KEYNOTE-052): a multicentre, single-arm, phase 2 study. Lancet Oncol. 2017;18(11):1483–92. https://doi.org/10.1016/S1470-2045(17)30616-2.

40. Passiglia F, et al. Looking for the best immune-checkpoint inhibitor in pre-treated NSCLC patients: an indirect comparison between nivolumab, pembrolizumab and atezolizumab. Int J Cancer. 2018; https://doi.org/10.1002/ijc.31136.

41. Rini BI, et al. Pembrolizumab plus axitinib versus sunitinib for advanced renal-cell carcinoma. N Engl J Med. 2019;380(12):1116–27. https://doi.org/10.1056/NEJMoa1816714.

42. Plimack ER, et al. Pembrolizumab plus axitinib versus sunitinib as first-line therapy for advanced renal cell carcinoma (RCC): Updated analysis of KEYNOTE-426. J Clin Oncol. 2020;38(15_suppl):5001. https://doi.org/10.1200/JCO.2020.38.15_suppl.5001.

43. Fuchs CS, et al. Safety and efficacy of pembrolizumab monotherapy in patients with previously treated advanced gastric and gastroesophageal junction cancer: phase 2 clinical KEYNOTE-059 trial. JAMA Oncol. 2018;4(5):e180013. https://doi.org/10.1001/jamaoncol.2018.0013.

44. Shitara K, et al. Efficacy and safety of pembrolizumab or pembrolizumab plus chemotherapy vs chemotherapy alone for patients with first-line, advanced gastric cancer: the KEYNOTE-062 phase 3 randomized clinical trial. JAMA Oncol. 2020;6(10):1571–80. https://doi.org/10.1001/jamaoncol.2020.3370.
45. Kojima T, et al. Randomized phase III KEYNOTE-181 study of pembrolizumab versus chemotherapy in advanced esophageal cancer. J Clin Oncol Off J Am Soc Clin Oncol. 2020;38(35):4138–48. https://doi.org/10.1200/JCO.20.01888.
46. Shah MA, et al. Efficacy and safety of pembrolizumab for heavily pretreated patients with advanced, metastatic adenocarcinoma or squamous cell carcinoma of the esophagus: the phase 2 KEYNOTE-180 study. JAMA Oncol. 2019;5(4):546–50. https://doi.org/10.1001/jamaoncol.2018.5441.
47. Kato K. Abstract LBA8_PR "pembrolizumab plus chemotherapy versus chemotherapy as first-line therapy in patients with advanced esophageal cancer: the phase 3 KEYNOTE-590 study" will be presented by Ken Kato during the Presidential Symposium III on Monday, 21 Septe. Ann Oncol. 2020;31(4):S1142–S1215. https://doi.org/10.1016/annonc/annonc32569.
48. Zhu AX, et al. Pembrolizumab in patients with advanced hepatocellular carcinoma previously treated with sorafenib (KEYNOTE-224): a non-randomised, open-label phase 2 trial. Lancet Oncol. 2018;19(7):940–52. https://doi.org/10.1016/S1470-2045(18)30351-6.
49. Seiwert TY, et al. Safety and clinical activity of pembrolizumab for treatment of recurrent or metastatic squamous cell carcinoma of the head and neck (KEYNOTE-012): an open-label, multicentre, phase 1b trial. Lancet Oncol. 2016;17(7):956–65. https://doi.org/10.1016/S1470-2045(16)30066-3.
50. Le DT, et al. Phase II open-label study of pembrolizumab in treatment-refractory, microsatellite instability-high/mismatch repair-deficient metastatic colorectal cancer: KEYNOTE-164. J Clin Oncol Off J Am Soc Clin Oncol. 2020;38(1):11–9. https://doi.org/10.1200/JCO.19.02107.
51. Marabelle A, et al. Efficacy of pembrolizumab in patients with noncolorectal high microsatellite instability/mismatch repair-deficient cancer: results from the phase II KEYNOTE-158 study. J Clin Oncol Off J Am Soc Clin Oncol. 2020;38(1):1–10. https://doi.org/10.1200/JCO.19.02105.
52. André T, et al. Pembrolizumab in microsatellite-instability-high advanced colorectal cancer. N Engl J Med. 2020;383(23):2207–18. https://doi.org/10.1056/NEJMoa2017699.
53. Forster MD, Devlin M-J. Immune checkpoint inhibition in head and neck cancer. Front Oncol. 2018;8:310. [Online]. Available: https://www.frontiersin.org/article/10.3389/fonc.2018.00310
54. Muro K, et al. Pembrolizumab for patients with PD-L1-positive advanced gastric cancer (KEYNOTE-012): a multicentre, open-label, phase 1b trial. Lancet Oncol. 2016;17(6):717–26. https://doi.org/10.1016/S1470-2045(16)00175-3.
55. Burtness B, et al. Pembrolizumab alone or with chemotherapy versus cetuximab with chemotherapy for recurrent or metastatic squamous cell carcinoma of the head and neck (KEYNOTE-048): a randomised, open-label, phase 3 study. Lancet (London, England). 2019;394(10212):1915–28. https://doi.org/10.1016/S0140-6736(19)32591-7.
56. Weber J, et al. Adjuvant nivolumab versus ipilimumab in resected stage III or IV melanoma. N Engl J Med. 2017;377(19):1824–35. https://doi.org/10.1056/NEJMoa1709030.
57. Robert C, et al. Nivolumab in previously untreated melanoma without BRAF mutation. N Engl J Med. 2015;372(4):320–30. https://doi.org/10.1056/NEJMoa1412082.
58. Larkin J, et al. Five-year survival with combined nivolumab and ipilimumab in advanced melanoma. N Engl J Med. 2019;381(16):1535–46. https://doi.org/10.1056/NEJMoa1910836.
59. Wolchok JD, et al. Overall survival with combined nivolumab and ipilimumab in advanced melanoma. N Engl J Med. 2017;377(14):1345–56. https://doi.org/10.1056/NEJMoa1709684.
60. Brahmer J, et al. Nivolumab versus docetaxel in advanced squamous-cell non–small-cell lung cancer. N Engl J Med. 2015;373(2):123–35. https://doi.org/10.1056/NEJMoa1504627.
61. Hellmann MD, et al. Nivolumab plus ipilimumab in advanced non-small-cell lung cancer. N Engl J Med. 2019; https://doi.org/10.1056/NEJMoa1910231.
62. Motzer RJ, et al. Avelumab plus axitinib versus sunitinib for advanced renal-cell carcinoma. N Engl J Med. 2019;380(12):1103–15. https://doi.org/10.1056/NEJMoa1816047.

63. Kato K, et al. Nivolumab versus chemotherapy in patients with advanced oesophageal squamous cell carcinoma refractory or intolerant to previous chemotherapy (ATTRACTION-3): a multicentre, randomised, open-label, phase 3 trial. Lancet Oncol. 2019;20(11):1506–17. https://doi.org/10.1016/S1470-2045(19)30626-6.

64. Overman MJ, et al. Nivolumab in patients with metastatic DNA mismatch repair-deficient or microsatellite instability-high colorectal cancer (CheckMate 142): an open-label, multicentre, phase 2 study. Lancet Oncol. 2017;18(9):1182–91. https://doi.org/10.1016/S1470-2045(17)30422-9.

65. Rittmeyer A, et al. Atezolizumab versus docetaxel in patients with previously treated non-small-cell lung cancer (OAK): a phase 3, open-label, multicentre randomised controlled trial. Lancet. 2017;389(10066):255–65. https://doi.org/10.1016/S0140-6736(16)32517-X.

66. Fehrenbacher L, et al. Atezolizumab versus docetaxel for patients with previously treated non-small-cell lung cancer (POPLAR): a multicentre, open-label, phase 2 randomised controlled trial. Lancet (London, England). 2016;387(10030):1837–46. https://doi.org/10.1016/S0140-6736(16)00587-0.

67. West H, et al. Atezolizumab in combination with carboplatin plus nab-paclitaxel chemotherapy compared with chemotherapy alone as first-line treatment for metastatic non-squamous non-small-cell lung cancer (IMpower130): a multicentre, randomised, open-label, phase 3 tria. Lancet Oncol. 2019; https://doi.org/10.1016/S1470-2045(19)30167-6.

68. Socinski MA, et al. Atezolizumab for first-line treatment of metastatic nonsquamous NSCLC. N Engl J Med. 2018; https://doi.org/10.1056/NEJMoa1716948.

69. Reinmuth N, et al. Impower110: interim os analysis of a phase III study of atezolizumab (ATEZO) vs platinum-based chemotherapy (chemo) as 1l treatment (tx) in pd-l1-selected NSCLC. Ann Oncol. 2019;30(Suppl 5):v851–v934.

70. Horn L, et al. First-line atezolizumab plus chemotherapy in extensive-stage small-cell lung cancer. N Engl J Med. 2018;379(23):2220–9. https://doi.org/10.1056/NEJMoa1809064.

71. Finn RS, et al. Atezolizumab plus bevacizumab in unresectable hepatocellular carcinoma. N Engl J Med. 2020;382(20):1894–905. https://doi.org/10.1056/NEJMoa1915745.

72. Schmid P, et al. Atezolizumab and nab-paclitaxel in advanced triple-negative breast cancer. N Engl J Med. 2018;379(22):2108–21. https://doi.org/10.1056/NEJMoa1809615.

73. Powles T, et al. Avelumab maintenance therapy for advanced or metastatic urothelial carcinoma. N Engl J Med. 2020;383(13):1218–30. https://doi.org/10.1056/NEJMoa2002788.

74. Antonia SJ, et al. overall survival with durvalumab after chemoradiotherapy in stage III NSCLC. N Engl J Med. 2018;379(24):2342–50. https://doi.org/10.1056/NEJMoa1809697.

75. Faivre-Finn C, et al. Four-year survival with durvalumab after chemoradiotherapy in stage III NSCLC: an update From the PACIFIC trial. J Thorac Oncol. 2021;16(5):860–7. https://doi.org/10.1016/j.jtho.2020.12.015.

76. Paz-Ares LG, et al. Durvalumab ± tremelimumab + platinum-etoposide in first-line extensive-stage SCLC (ES-SCLC): Updated results from the phase III CASPIAN study. J Clin Oncol. 2020;38(15_suppl):9002. https://doi.org/10.1200/JCO.2020.38.15_suppl.9002.

77. Schadendorf D, et al. Health-related quality of life results from the phase III CheckMate 067 study. Eur J Cancer. 2017;82:80–91. https://doi.org/10.1016/j.ejca.2017.05.031.

78. Eggermont AMM, et al. Adjuvant ipilimumab versus placebo after complete resection of high-risk stage III melanoma (EORTC 18071): a randomised, double-blind, phase 3 trial. Lancet Oncol. 2015;16(5):522–30. https://doi.org/10.1016/S1470-2045(15)70122-1.

79. Lonardi S, et al. A2 – Combination of nivolumab (nivo) + ipilimumab (ipi) in the treatment of patients (pts) with deficient DNA mismatch repair (dMMR)/high microsatellite instability (MSI-H) metastatic colorectal cancer (mCRC): CheckMate 142 Study. Ann Oncol. 2017;28:vi3. https://doi.org/10.1093/annonc/mdx422.001.

Alessandro Inno and Stefania Gori

Introduction

Immunotherapy has a peculiar toxicity profile characterized by immune-related adverse events (irAEs) that can potentially affect any organ or system, including the cardiovascular system [1, 2]. Cardiovascular irAEs have been probably under-recognized until 2016, when two cases of fulminant myocarditis associated with immune checkpoint inhibitors (ICIs) were reported [3]. Since then, the awareness as well as the reporting of immune-related myocarditis have increased [4, 5]. It is now acknowledged that not only the myocardium but also all the other parts of the cardiovascular system including pericardium, electrical circuits, and vessels can be affected by irAEs [6, 7].

In this chapter, clinical pictures of the main cardiovascular irAEs are summarized.

Myocarditis

Immune-related myocarditis is the most clinically relevant cardiovascular toxicity of immunotherapy. Although it is rare with an incidence rate ranging from 0.27% to 1.14% [3, 8], it is burdened by high mortality with a fatality rate of approximately 40–50% [9, 10]. Median time to onset is 30 days (interquartile range 18–60) as reported by a retrospective pharmacovigilance study, even if early cases occurring within 2 weeks after the first infusion of ICIs as well as late cases occurring ≥90 days have been also reported [3, 11]. Dual blockade with anti-CTLA4 and anti-PD1 antibodies seems to be associated with higher risk of immune-related myocarditis

A. Inno · S. Gori (✉)
Medical Oncology, IRCCS Ospedale Sacro Cuore Don Calabria,
Negrar di Valpolicella, Verona, Italy
e-mail: alessandro.inno@sacrocuore.it; stefania.gori@sacrocuore.it

© The Author(s), under exclusive license to Springer Nature
Switzerland AG 2022

25

A. Russo et al. (eds.), *Cardio-Oncology*, Current Clinical Pathology,
https://doi.org/10.1007/978-3-030-97744-3_3

(incidence up to 2.4%), earlier onset, more severe presentation, and increased mortality as compared with single-agent ICIs [3, 10].

Immune-related pericardial disease may have variable clinical presentation including nonspecific complaints of malaise, chest pain, shortness of breath, acute heart failure, pulmonary edema and, in severe cases, cardiogenic shock, multiorgan failure, heart block, and both atrial and ventricular arrhythmias leading to death [6, 7, 12, 13]. Myocarditis may also be associated with other irAEs, mainly myositis or myasthenia gravis [10]. Although myocarditis is generally symptomatic and severe or life-threatening, some cases of smoldering myocarditis in the form of asymptomatic or pauci-symptomatic elevation of cardiac biomarkers have been also reported, but the clinical significance of this entity remains unclear [14]. In the absence of symptoms, isolated elevation of troponin is not sufficient to define myocarditis according to the National Cancer Institute, Common Terminology Criteria for Adverse Events (NCI-CTCAE) version 5.0 [15].

Serum cardiac biomarkers such as troponin and creatine kinase-muscle/brain (CK-MB) armmunotherapy adverse evene almost always elevated, and the degree of troponin elevation seems to be associated with the risk of major complications and death [8]. Most patients have ECG abnormalities including intraventricular conduction delay, PR interval prolongation, and eventually complete heart block or several forms of arrhythmia [7, 8]. Echocardiography may show changes in cardiac chambers, geometry, or regional wall motion abnormalities [7], but approximately half of the patients do not develop a significant reduction in left ventricular ejection fraction (LVEF) [8]. Cardiac magnetic resonance imaging (MRI) is superior to echocardiography when myocarditis is suspected, being able to detect myocardial edema, necrosis, and scar formation [7]. Additionally, ^{18}F-FDG PET/CT can show active myocardial inflammation. When endomyocardial biopsy is available, pathology examination may reveal lymphocytic or macrophage infiltration of the myocardium [3, 7].

Noninflammatory Myocardial Dysfunction

Immunotherapy may also lead to heart failure without associated myocarditis, through noninflammatory forms of myocardial dysfunction including dilated cardiomyopathy with global left ventricular impairment and Takotsubo syndrome [6, 12].

Dilated cardiomyopathy presents with new global ventricular dysfunction in the absence of increase in cardiac troponin, no cardiac MRI or ^{18}F-FDG PET/CT evidence of active myocardial inflammation, and no inflammatory cell infiltrate on endomyocardial biopsy [6].

Takotsubo syndrome presents with acute heart failure associated with regional wall motion abnormalities involving the apical and mid-left ventricular myocardium, unobstructed coronary arteries, BNP elevation, and acquired long-QT syndrome, with no signs of active myocarditis at cardiac MRI, ^{18}F-FDG PET/CT, or endomyocardial biopsy [6, 16].

Arrhythmias

Treatment with ICIs may be complicated by atrial fibrillation (AF), atrioventricular (AV) block, ventricular arrhythmias, and, in severe cases, sudden death from complete heart block [17].

A systematic review published in 2018 reported that AV block and ventricular arrhythmias occurred respectively in 10% and 5–10% of patients with ICI-related cardiovascular adverse events and were associated with high mortality [18]. AV block and other conduction disorders might be secondary to myocarditis with an inflammatory infiltration of the AV nodal area or the conduction system. Similarly, ventricular arrhythmias might be caused by myocarditis or other cardiomyopathies caused by ICIs. The new onset of conduction disorders or ventricular arrhythmias is generally associated with a more complicated clinical course of immune-related cardiac toxicity and should prompt the diagnostic workup for myocarditis [17].

AF has been reported in patients treated with CAR T cells or ICIs [17, 19]. It could be induced by an increased general inflammatory status due to immunotherapy, as well as by immune-related pericarditis, cardiomyopathy, or thyroid dysfunction [17].

Pericardial Disease

Immune-related pericardial disease may occur in the form of pericarditis (with or without associated myocarditis), pericardial effusion, or pericardial tamponade [6, 7]. The exact incidence of pericardial toxicity is not completely known, probably because of the initial under-recognition of this event as an irAE. In a retrospective study on 2830 patients treated with ICIs, pericardial toxicity was uncommon with an incidence rate of approximately 0.1% [20]. However, immune-related pericardial disease may be more frequent among specific populations, such as patients with lung cancer treated with anti-PD1 antibodies that have an incidence rate exceeding 6% in some series [10, 21]. Although reversible in the majority of cases, a fatality rate of approximately 20% has been reported by a pharmacovigilance study [10]. Median time to onset is 30 days (interquartile range 9–90), although cases of late toxicity occurred even more than 1 year after starting ICIs were also described [10, 22, 23].

Clinical presentation may include chest pain relieved by forward position, hypotension, dyspnea, muffled heart sounds, jugular vein distension, new or worsening pericardial effusion at echocardiography or CT scan, cardiomegaly at chest X-ray, ECG alterations including new PR depression and diffuse saddle-shaped ST elevation, and/or pericardial inflammation at cardiac MRI and ^{18}F-FDG PET/CT [7, 24]. In about one-third of cases, acute inflammatory cells are found in pericardial effusion cytology examinations [24]. When available, pericardial biopsy may reveal fibrinous pericarditis with lymphocytic infiltrate, but other pathology findings have been described, including pericardial hyperplasia and nonspecific acute or chronic pericardial inflammation, with or without myocardial involvement [25–28].

In most of the reported cases, ICI-associated pericardial disease was severe [10], often with tamponade physiology requiring pericardiocentesis, surgical drainage, or pericardial window. A retrospective, mono-institutional study showed that, although the incidence of pericardial disease among cancer patients receiving ICIs was low (0.38%), the need for pericardiocentesis was higher compared to cancer patients not treated with ICIs, with a relative risk of 3.1 [24], but the reason for this increased need for pericardiocentesis remains unclear.

Vasculitis

Immune-related vasculitis can potentially affect vessels of any size, but it affects more frequently large vessels mainly in the form of temporal arteritis or aortitis [7]. Particularly, a pharmacovigilance study published in 2018 reported an overreporting of temporal arteritis among patients treated with ICIs compared to patients not treated with ICIs [10]. In this study, temporal arteritis was more frequently reported with anti-CTLA4 than with anti-PD1 or anti-PDL1 antibodies. The median time to onset was 21 days (interquartile range 21–98) for temporal arteritis and 55 days (interquartile range 21–98) for vasculitis overall. Whereas no deaths were specifically reported for patients with immune-related temporal arteritis, the fatality rate was 6% for vasculitis overall [10].

Temporal arteritis is a disorder characterized by inflammation of the aorta and its branches, presenting with headache, jaw claudication, transient monocular visual loss (amaurosis fugax) or diplopia, and systemic symptoms such as fatigue, fever, and weight loss [7]. Visual impairment has been reported in 28% of patients with immune-related temporal arteritis [10]. Patients have generally high levels of inflammatory markers such as erythrocyte sedimentation rate and C-reactive protein. A biopsy of the temporal artery usually demonstrates granulomas consisting of T cells and macrophages.

Myocardial Infarction

Myocardial infarction has been reported during treatment with ICIs [6, 29]. It should be considered that patients with cancer may also have overt or subclinical cardiovascular disease with underlying risk factors for myocardial infarction. Therefore this event could be not related to immunotherapy only, but more probably, it is often the result of a multifactorial process. However, emerging data demonstrate that treatment with ICIs increases the risk of myocardial infarction.

In a matched cohort study including 2842 cancer patients treated with ICIs and 2842 cancer patients not treated with ICIs, the incidence of myocardial infarction in patients receiving immunotherapy was approximately 2% [30]. In a multivariable model which included known cardiovascular risk factors, ICIs were associated with a significantly higher risk for cardiovascular events including myocardial infarction, revascularization, and ischemic stroke (hazard ratio 4.50, 95% CI 3.30–6.13).

Interestingly, there was an increasing incidence of myocardial infarction in the 2-year period after ICIs as compared with the 2-year period before ICIs (hazard ratio 4.84, 95% CI 2.76–8.09). The increased risk of cardiovascular events associated with ICIs seems to be related to the accelerated progression of atherosclerosis [30]. However, other mechanisms cannot be excluded, since a case of coronary spasm during treatment with anti-PD1 antibodies has been described [29].

Myocardial infarction usually presents with chest pain, new ECG ischemic abnormalities including ST elevation, ST depression, or T-wave inversion, cardiac troponin elevation, and usually new regional wall motion abnormalities on echocardiogram or cardiac MRI [6]. Differential diagnosis includes coronary vasculitis and focal myocarditis [30, 31]. The gold standard for diagnosis is coronarography, and percutaneous coronary intervention is indicated in cases of hemodynamically significant stenosis [6].

References

1. Inno A, Metro G, Bironzo P, Grimaldi AM, Grego E, Nunno VD, Picasso V, Massari F, Gori S. Pathogenesis, clinical manifestations and management of immune checkpoint inhibitors toxicity. Tumori. 2017; https://doi.org/10.5301/tj.5000625.
2. Champiat S, Lambotte O, Barreau E, et al. Management of immune checkpoint blockade dysimmune toxicities: a collaborative position paper. Ann Oncol. 2016;27:559–74.
3. Johnson DB, Balko JM, Compton ML, et al. Fulminant myocarditis with combination immune checkpoint blockade. N Engl J Med. 2016;375:1749–55.
4. Moslehi JJ, Salem JE, Sosman JA, Lebrun-Vignes B, Johnson DB. Increased reporting of fatal immune checkpoint inhibitor-associated myocarditis. Lancet. 2018;391:933.
5. Varricchi G, Galdiero MR, Mercurio V, Bonaduce D, Marone G, Tocchetti CG. Pharmacovigilating cardiotoxicity of immune checkpoint inhibitors. Lancet Oncol. 2018;19:1545–6.
6. Lyon AR, Yousaf N, Battisti NML, Moslehi J, Larkin J. Immune checkpoint inhibitors and cardiovascular toxicity. Lancet Oncol. 2018; https://doi.org/10.1016/S1470-2045(18)30457-1.
7. Hu JR, Florido R, Lipson EJ, Naidoo J, Ardehali R, Tocchetti CG, Lyon AR, Padera RF, Johnson DB, Moslehi J. Cardiovascular toxicities associated with immune checkpoint inhibitors. Cardiovasc Res. 2019;115:854–68.
8. Mahmood SS, Fradley MG, Cohen JV, et al. Myocarditis in patients treated with immune checkpoint inhibitors. J Am Coll Cardiol. 2018;71:1755–64.
9. Wang DY, Salem JE, Cohen JV, et al. Fatal toxic effects associated with immune checkpoint inhibitors: a systematic review and meta-analysis. JAMA Oncol. 2018;4:1721–8.
10. Salem JE, Manouchehri A, Moey M, et al. Cardiovascular toxicities associated with immune checkpoint inhibitors: an observational, retrospective, pharmacovigilance study. Lancet Oncol. 2018;19:1579–89.
11. Dolladille C, Ederhy S, Allouche S, et al. Late cardiac adverse events in patients with cancer treated with immune checkpoint inhibitors. J Immunother Cancer. 2020;8:1–10.
12. Yang S, Asnani A. Cardiotoxicities associated with immune checkpoint inhibitors. Curr Probl Cancer. 2018;42:422–32.
13. Ganatra S, Neilan TG. Immune checkpoint inhibitor-associated myocarditis. Oncologist. 2018;23:879–86.
14. Norwood TG, Westbrook BC, Johnson DB, Litovsky SH, Terry NL, McKee SB, Gertler AS, Moslehi JJ, Conry RM. Smoldering myocarditis following immune checkpoint blockade. J Immunother Cancer. 2017;5:4–9.

15. Cancer Institute N. Common terminology criteria for adverse events (CTCAE) common terminology criteria for adverse events (CTCAE) v5.0. 2017. https://ctep.cancer.gov/protocoldevelopment/electronic_applications/ctc.htm.
16. Geisler BP, Raad RA, Esaian D, Sharon E, Schwartz DR. Apical ballooning and cardiomyopathy in a melanoma patient treated with ipilimumab: a case of takotsubo-like syndrome. J Immunother Cancer. 2015; https://doi.org/10.1186/s40425-015-0048-2.
17. Herrmann J. Adverse cardiac effects of cancer therapies: cardiotoxicity and arrhythmia. Nat Rev Cardiol. 2020; https://doi.org/10.1038/s41569-020-0348-1.
18. Mir H, Alhussein M, Alrashidi S, Alzayer H, Alshatti A, Valettas N, Mukherjee SD, Nair V, Leong DP. Cardiac complications associated with checkpoint inhibition: a systematic review of the literature in an important emerging area. Can J Cardiol. 2018;34:1059–68.
19. Brudno JN, Kochenderfer JN. Toxicities of chimeric antigen receptor T cells: recognition and management. Blood. 2016;127:3321–30.
20. Chahine J, Collier P, Maroo A, Tang WHW, Klein AL. Myocardial and pericardial toxicity associated with immune checkpoint inhibitors in cancer patients. JACC: Case Rep. 2020;2:191–9.
21. Canale ML, Camerini A, Casolo G, et al. Incidence of pericardial effusion in patients with advanced non-small cell lung cancer receiving immunotherapy. Adv Ther. 2020; https://doi.org/10.1007/s12325-020-01386-y.
22. Oristrell G, Bañeras J, Ros J, Muñoz E. Cardiac tamponade and adrenal insufficiency due to pembrolizumab: a case report. Eur Heart J – Case Rep. 2018; https://doi.org/10.1093/ehjcr/yty038.
23. Anastasia S, Audrey ML, Jennifer A, Constance T, Mariana M, François G, Stéphane O, Laurence W. Pericardial effusion under nivolumab: case-reports and review of the literature. J Immunother Cancer. 2019; https://doi.org/10.1186/s40425-019-0760-4.
24. Palaskas N, Morgan J, Daigle T, et al. Targeted cancer therapies with pericardial effusions requiring pericardiocentesis focusing on immune checkpoint inhibitors. Am J Cardiol. 2019;123:1351–7.
25. Altan M, Toki MI, Gettinger SN, Carvajal-Hausdorf DE, Zugazagoitia J, Sinard JH, Herbst RS, Rimm DL. Immune checkpoint inhibitor–associated pericarditis. J Thorac Oncol. 2019;14:1102–8.
26. de Almeida DVP, Gomes JR, Haddad FJ, Buzaid AC. Immune-mediated pericarditis with pericardial tamponade during nivolumab therapy. J Immunother. 2018;41:329–31.
27. Nesfeder J, Elsensohn AN, Thind M, Lennon J, Domsky S. Pericardial effusion with tamponade physiology induced by nivolumab. Int J Cardiol. 2016;222:613–4.
28. Yun S, Vincelette ND, Mansour I, Hariri D, Motamed S. Late onset ipilimumab-induced pericarditis and pericardial effusion: a rare but life threatening complication. Case Rep Oncol Med. 2015;2015:1–5.
29. Nykl R, Fischer O, Vykoupil K, Taborsky M. A unique reason for coronary spasm causing temporary ST elevation myocardial infarction (inferior STEMI) – systemic inflammatory response syndrome after use of pembrolizumab. Arch Med Sci – Atherosc Dis. 2017; https://doi.org/10.5114/amsad.2017.72531.
30. Drobni ZD, Alvi RM, Taron J, et al. Association between immune checkpoint inhibitors with cardiovascular events and atherosclerotic plaque. Circulation. 2020; https://doi.org/10.1161/circulationaha.120.049981.
31. Novo G, Di Lisi D, Manganaro R, et al. Arterial stiffness: effects of anticancer drugs used for breast cancer women. Front Physiol. 2021;12:661464. Published 2021 May 13. https://doi.org/10.3389/fphys.2021.661464.

Pathophysiology of Cardiac Toxicity

4

Dimitrios Farmakis

Pathophysiology of Cardiac Toxicity: An Overview

Cardiotoxicity of anticancer therapy, including systemically acting drugs and radiotherapy, may practically include every known form of cardiovascular (CV) disease affecting the myocardium, endocardium and pericardium as well as the systemic and pulmonary circulation [1]. This broad range of manifestations results from the fact that anticancer modalities may act directly or indirectly on every part of the CV system, either by causing cell dysfunction, necrosis or apoptosis or by inducing metabolic or other abnormalities. The effect of anticancer therapy on the CV system is further modified by its interaction with two additional factors, patient's comorbidities and risk factors and cancer itself (Fig. 4.1) [2, 3]. Demographic features, past history of CV disease, cardiac or extra-cardiac comorbidities, coexisting cardiometabolic and genetic factors may render the cancer patient more susceptible to toxicity from anticancer therapy [4, 5]. On the other hand, cancer itself may affect the CV system by invading directly the heart and vessels, by causing a prothrombotic state that increases the risk of thromboembolism or by inducing inflammation, cachexia and other metabolic or systemic abnormalities that may in turn affect CV function [2, 6]. In addition, recent evidence suggests that the interaction of cardiac and malignant cells with their extracellular environment may mediate the progression of both heart disease and cancer [7].

D. Farmakis (✉)
University of Cyprus Medical School, Nicosia, Cyprus
e-mail: farmakis.dimitrios@ucy.ac.cy

A. Russo et al. (eds.), *Cardio-Oncology*, Current Clinical Pathology,
https://doi.org/10.1007/978-3-030-97744-3_4

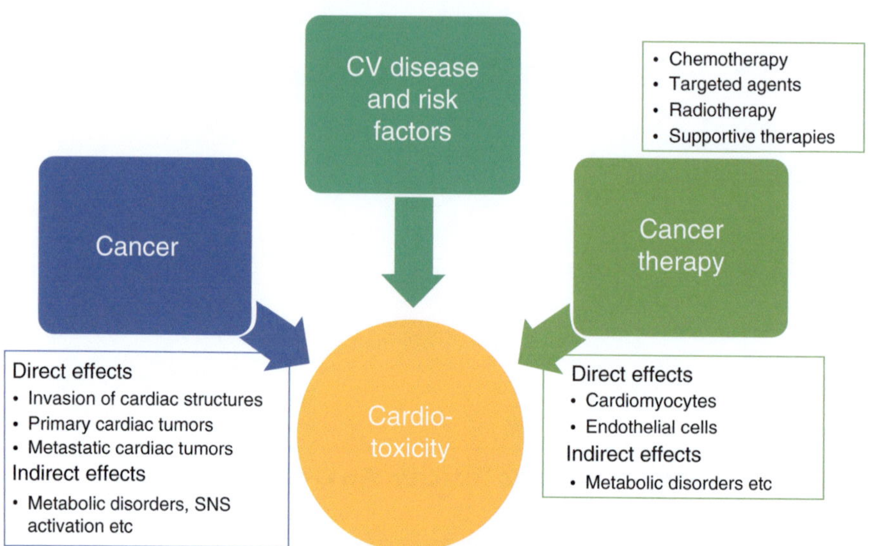

Fig. 4.1 Conceptual framework for the pathophysiology of cardiovascular toxicity in patients with cancer. (Reprinted with permission from Farmakis et al. [2])

Cardiac Dysfunction and Heart Failure

Anticancer therapy-induced cardiac dysfunction may range from asymptomatic left ventricular (LV) dysfunction to clinically manifested heart failure. Asymptomatic LV dysfunction may be subtle, detected only by serum biomarkers or sensitive imaging techniques, including high-sensitivity cardiac troponin (hs-cTn), natriuretic peptides and LV strain in deformation imaging, or more prominent, characterized by decreased LV ejection fraction (LVEF) [8, 9]. Symptomatic LV dysfunction may be manifested by typical HF symptoms such as dyspnoea, peripheral oedema or fatigue. However, these symptoms are often difficult to interpret as they may also be provoked by cancer.

Cardiac dysfunction may result from the direct toxic effect of anticancer therapy on cardiomyocytes (Fig. 4.2). It has previously been suggested that systematically acting anticancer drugs exerting toxic effect on cardiomyocytes may be categorized into two types according to whether the myocardial injury is reversible or not [10]. According to this classification, agents causing irreversible cardiomyocyte damage, leading to cell necrosis or apoptosis, are characterized as type I agents, while those causing potentially reversible cellular dysfunction are type II agents. Typical examples of type I and II drugs include anthracyclines and trastuzumab, respectively. The reversibility or not of myocardial injury at the cellular level may, however, be determined by additional factors, such as the interaction among anticancer drugs. For example, it has been suggested that the typical type II agent trastuzumab may potentiate anthracycline-induced cardiotoxicity when the two drugs are administered simultaneously, thus contributing to cardiac cell death [11].

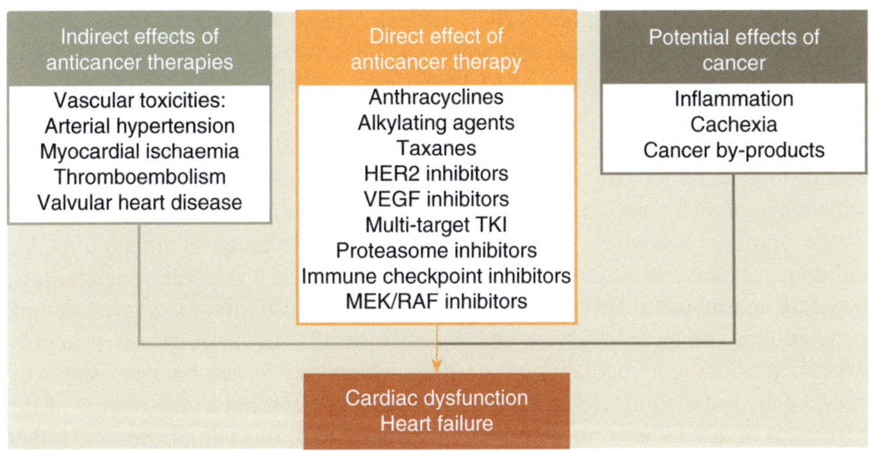

Fig. 4.2 Pathophysiology of cardiac dysfunction and heart failure in cancer patients receiving anticancer therapy

Anthracycline-induced cardiac dysfunction represents the prototype and the most intensively studied form of cardiotoxicity of anticancer drugs. Several mechanisms have been proposed for anthracycline-induced cardiac dysfunction. Anthracyclines intercalate into nucleic acids and induce oxidative stress through the production of reactive oxygen species that cause peroxidation of proteins, nucleic acids and lipids as well as inhibition of DNA and RNA synthesis and repair in cardiomyocytes. These changes lead in turn to sarcomere protein dysfunction, mitochondrial dysfunction and ultimately myocyte death [12]. More recently, it has been shown that topoisomerase 2β, an enzyme required for DNA transcription, replication and recombination, may play a key role in mediating anthracycline-induced cardiotoxicity by inducing DNA double-strand breaks and transcriptome damage; these changes lead in turn to the activation of the p53 apoptotic pathway, mitochondrial dysfunction and production of reactive oxygen species, causing cardiomyocyte dysfunction or death [13]. Additional proposed mechanisms for anthracycline-induced cardiotoxicity include alterations in multidrug resistance (MDR) efflux proteins, thus impairing cellular clearance capacity, leading to intracellular anthracycline accumulation and decreased activation of mesenchymal and circulating progenitor cells, thus impairing cardio-reparative capacity against stressors [12].

Human epidermal growth factor receptor (HER2/ErbB) inhibitors are either monoclonal antibodies (e.g. trastuzumab, pertuzumab) or TKI (e.g. lapatinib, neratinib) used mainly for the treatment of breast cancer overexpressing HER2. These drugs have been associated with cardiac dysfunction and heart failure, and they also increase the susceptibility of the heart to anthracycline-induced cardiotoxicity, as previously stressed. HER2 inhibitors interfere with the neuregulin-HER2/HER4 pathway that is responsible for cardiomyocyte growth, survival and homeostasis, as well as the cell response to stress. HER2 inhibition impairs the capacity of cardiomyocytes to respond favourably to different stressors, thus rendering the cells more susceptible to dysfunction or death [12].

Immune checkpoint inhibitors (ICI) are monoclonal antibodies directed against cytotoxic T-lymphocyte-associated protein 4 (CTLA-4) or programmed cell death protein 1 (PD-1) and its ligand (PD-L1) that are signalling molecules located on T lymphocytes and antigen-presenting cells suppressing their activity, thus allowing cancer cells to escape immune surveillance [14]. By inhibiting these regulators, ICI enhance the activity of the immune system, having considerable efficacy against a wide range of malignancies. Besides the antitumour effects, however, the activation of the immune system by ICI may also cause a wide range of immune-related inflammatory adverse events affecting various organs, such as colitis, pneumonitis, hepatitis and myositis [15]. In this context, ICI may also affect the myocardium, pericardium, conduction system and vasculature. ICI cardiotoxicity is primarily expressed as immune-mediated myocarditis, which may further be complicated by ventricular dysfunction, HF and arrhythmias [16]. According to the reports of the first cases of ICI-induced myocarditis, the incidence of this complication is rather low, up to 1%, but its mortality rate can be as high as 50% [17, 18]. Additional, immune-mediated CV complications of ICI may include pericarditis, vasculitis, Takotsubo and conduction system abnormalities [16].

Proteasome inhibitors, such as bortezomib and carfilzomib, are used for the treatment of multiple myeloma. These drugs block the action of the proteasome that is responsible for the degradation of dysfunctional or unnecessary proteins. The ubiquitin-proteasome system plays an important role in vascular homeostasis [19]. Proteasome inhibition results in the accumulation of dysfunctional proteins in different cells, including in endothelial cells, leading to CV toxicity expressed as arterial hypertension, cardiac dysfunction, heart failure, venous thromboembolism and thrombotic microangiopathy [20–22].

Small-molecule tyrosine kinase inhibitors (TKI), such as vascular endothelial growth factor inhibitors (VEGFi), addressed in detail later in this chapter, besides their well-known vascular toxicities, may also induce myocardial dysfunction. Cardiomyocytes may further be indirectly affected by the toxic effect of anticancer therapy on vascular and cardiac endothelial cells, discussed later in this chapter, through the cardiomyocyte-endothelial interaction. Other forms of cardiovascular toxicity, also discussed later in this chapter, including arterial or pulmonary hypertension, myocardial ischemia, arterial or venous thromboembolism and valvular disease, may further cause cardiac dysfunction and heart failure (Fig. 4.2). It has further been proposed that metabolic by-products produced by malignant cells, along with cancer-induced inflammatory reaction and cachexia, may further affect cardiac function [7].

The combination of MEK and RAF inhibitors (e.g. trametinib and dabrafenib), used for the treatment of malignant melanoma and non-small cell lung cancer, has been associated with an increased risk of cardiac dysfunction along with vascular toxicities, mainly arterial hypertension [23]. MEK inhibition, on the one hand, compromises the cardioprotective MEK/ERK pathway, while, on the other hand, it increases the cardiotoxic p38 MAP pathway, both having a negative impact on cardiac function [24, 25].

Vascular Disease

Vascular disease resulting from anticancer therapy may include arterial hypertension, coronary artery disease, pulmonary hypertension and arterial or venous thromboembolic events. The effect of many anticancer agents and radiotherapy on endothelial cell integrity and function holds a central role in the development of vascular toxicities [26].

The primary class of anticancer agents interfering with endothelial function are VEGFi. The VEGF protein family plays a crucial role in the homeostasis of the vascular system through the regulation of survival, proliferation and migration of endothelial cells. VEGF signalling activates intracellular second-messenger and pro-survival pathways, such as PI3K/Akt/mTOR and MAPK/ERK, and promotes NO synthesis [27]. VEGFi are monoclonal antibodies, such as bevacizumab, that inhibit circulating VEGF, or small-molecule TKI, such as sunitinib, sorafenib, pazopanib and vandetanib, that inhibit multiple tyrosine kinases involved in different pathways including VEGF, platelet-derived growth factor (PDGF) or c-Kit pathways. VEFGi are effective against a wide range of malignancies. However, VEGF inhibition impairs endothelial function, leading to reduce NO synthesis, impaired vasodilation, platelet activation, oxidative stress and inflammation, which may in turn result in multiple vascular toxicities, while may further contribute to myocardial dysfunction and heart failure [28, 29]. Inhibition of VEGF signalling may also promote endothelial dysfunction through the impairment of pericyte-endothelial cell interaction and the release of endothelial cell-derived microparticles (ECMP). Pericytes are perivascular cells in the microcirculation that interact with endothelial cells, the one affecting the survival and function of the other through VEGF and PDGF signalling, thus contributing to the homeostasis of the vasculature [30]. This interaction may be impaired by anticancer agents inhibiting both VEGF and PDGF such as sunitinib, sorafenib and pazopanib [31]. On the other hand, ECMP are vesicles cleaved by dysfunctional endothelial cells that promote inflammation and oxidative stress, impair NO synthesis and contribute to cell senescence [32].

VEGFi are typically associated with arterial hypertension, as well as arterial and venous thromboembolic events and cardiac dysfunction [26]. Arterial hypertension seems to result from an increase in vascular resistance and rarefaction [33]. Thromboembolic events are related to hypercoagulability and microvascular injury resulting from endothelial dysfunction [34]. Cardiac dysfunction has been attributed to the impaired ability of the heart to adapt to pressure overload and other types of stress and to regulate microvasculature growth in proportion to cardiomyocyte metabolic and growth changes; in addition, multi-target TKIs may further cause mitochondrial injury and apoptosis in cardiomyocytes [12, 35, 36].

Another class of targeted anticancer agents that may affect endothelial function and cause vascular toxicities are the Bcr-Abl inhibitors, used for the treatment of Philadelphia chromosome-positive chronic myeloid leukaemia. Bcr-Abl1 protein is a fusion protein produced by a chimeric gene created during DNA translocation. The Abl family of kinases seem to hold a role in endothelial cell survival and function through the AP-1/Tie2 pro-survival signalling pathway; thus, their inhibition may promote endothelial dysfunction [37]. Bcr-Abl inhibitors have been associated with a range of CV toxicities, including cardiac dysfunction (imatinib), arterial hypertension, angina, acute coronary syndrome, stroke, venous thromboembolism, peripheral arterial disease (nilotinib and ponatinib), and pulmonary hypertension (dasatinib) [26, 38, 39].

In what concerns chemotherapeutic agents, antimetabolites, such as 5-fluorouracil (5-FU) and capecitabine, have been associated with angina-following ST-segment/T-wave electrocardiographic changes. Coronary vasospasm leading to acute coronary syndrome (ACS) is typically associated with 5-FU administration. Besides vasospasm and related to endothelial injury and oxidative stress, additional pathogenetic mechanisms have been proposed including increased metabolic demands and impaired oxygen transfer capacity of red blood cells [40].

Another class of chemotherapeutic agents associated with vascular toxicity are platinum compounds, such as cisplatin. Cisplatin has been associated with not only acute coronary thrombosis but also late coronary events, for which other CV risk factors may hold a key role [41]. In terms of pathophysiology, it has been shown that cisplatin administration is followed by increase in markers of endothelial function such as intracellular adhesion molecule-1, tissue-type plasminogen activator, plasminogen activator inhibitor type 1 and von Willebrand factor, along with impaired flow-mediated dilatation and increased carotid intima-media thickness [42]. These adverse endothelial effects are prolonged as platinum compounds are measurable in the serum several years after chemotherapy, which may partly explain the late vascular toxicity observed in patients treated with these agents [43].

Chest irradiation may cause acute, subacute or late CV toxicities when parts of the heart and great vessels are included in the radiation field [44]. Radiation induces DNA injury that activates p53 and other pathways resulting in endothelial cell apoptosis or senescence, a process of accelerated cell ageing, while it also induces vascular inflammation, oxidative stress and hypercoagulability [45]. Chest irradiation has thus been associated with vascular degeneration and accelerated atherosclerosis, resulting in coronary artery disease, manifested years after radiotherapy [46].

In addition to anticancer therapies, endothelial dysfunction associated with patients' comorbidities such as diabetes mellitus, chronic kidney disease or systemic inflammatory conditions also contributes to vascular toxicities, rendering the patients more susceptible to vascular complications.

Among vascular toxicities, thromboembolism is probably the most important complication of cancer and its therapy as it represents the second leading cause of death in patients with malignancies, following cancer progression [47]. Cancer-associated thromboembolism results from the interaction of three main factors, the prothrombotic properties of cancer, the hypercoagulability associated with certain anticancer therapies and patient's risk factors. Cancer cells are known to cause direct activation of coagulation factors through the expression of tissue factors and the release of microparticles also expressing the tissue factor and cancer procoagulant factor, as well as indirect activation of coagulation pathways and platelets and inhibition of anticoagulant pathways and fibrinolysis through a systemic inflammatory reaction [48]. Specific tumour characteristics are also associated with an increased risk of thromboembolic complications, including the primary site (e.g. pancreas, stomach, ovaries, brain, lung, myeloma), the histological type (adenocarcinomas), genetic characteristics (e.g. JAK2 or K-ras mutations) and the advanced stage [49]. Anticancer therapy may further promote a hypercoagulable state through endothelial cell damage and induction of inflammatory reaction; cancer therapies associated with an increased risk of thromboembolism include platinum compounds, VEGFi, immune modulators such as thalidomide and lenalidomide, proteasome inhibitors, hormonal therapies and supportive therapies such as erythropoietin-stimulating agents [49]. In addition, cancer surgery and hospitalization also increase the risk of thromboembolism. Finally, patient-related thromboembolic risk factors include advanced age, female gender, obesity, a past history of thromboembolism, comorbid conditions, inherited coagulation defects, poor performance status and prolonged bed rest. It should also be stressed that cancer has been associated with atrial fibrillation, as described in detail below, that may in turn increase the risk of ischaemic stroke and systemic thromboembolism (Fig. 4.3) [6]. A combination of the above risk factors can lead to increased blood stasis, endothelial injury and hypercoagulability, thus fulfilling the triad of Virchow (Fig. 4.4) [50].

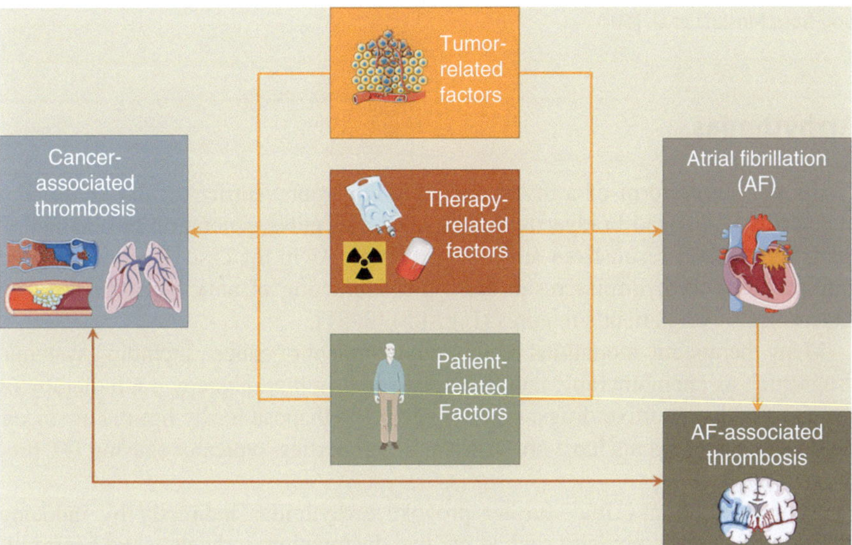

Fig. 4.3 Pathophysiology of cancer-associated thrombosis. Tumour characteristics, anticancer cancer and patient risk factors may increase the risk of thromboembolism, leading to cancer-associated thrombosis. In addition, cancer is often associated with atrial fibrillation, which further increases the risk of stroke and systemic thromboembolism

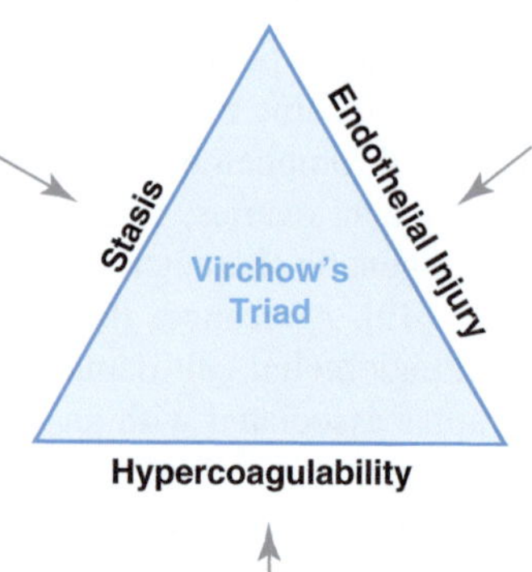

Fig. 4.4 Pathophysiology of thrombosis in cancer. A combination of thromboembolic risk factors related to the tumour, anticancer therapy and the patient may cause increased blood stasis, endothelial injury and hypercoagulability, thus fulfilling the triad of Virchow. (Reprinted with permission from Mosarla et al. [50])

Arrhythmias

Practically every form of arrhythmias including supraventricular and ventricular tachyarrhythmias and bradyarrhythmias related to pulse generation or conduction disturbances may result from anticancer therapy. As in the case of other forms of cardiotoxicity, arrhythmias result from the interaction of anticancer therapy and cancer itself with patient's features (Fig. 4.5) [3, 51].

Many therapeutic modalities used in the treatment of cancer, including systemic drugs such as chemotherapy, targeted agents and immunotherapy, radiotherapy of the chest and supportive drugs, may induce or predispose to rhythm disturbances. Some anticancer agents have pro-arrhythmic properties, typically causing QT prolongation [51].

Anticancer therapy may further provoke arrhythmias indirectly by inducing other forms of cardiotoxicity such as cardiac dysfunction, ischaemia and heart failure or by causing electrolyte and metabolic abnormalities resulting from gastrointestinal or other forms of toxicity [3]. Cancer itself may provoke or predispose to rhythm disturbances through the direct invasion of cardiac structures by a primary neoplasm or, more often, a metastatic tumour or through more systemic actions such as inflammation or autonomic nervous system imbalance. Finally, several

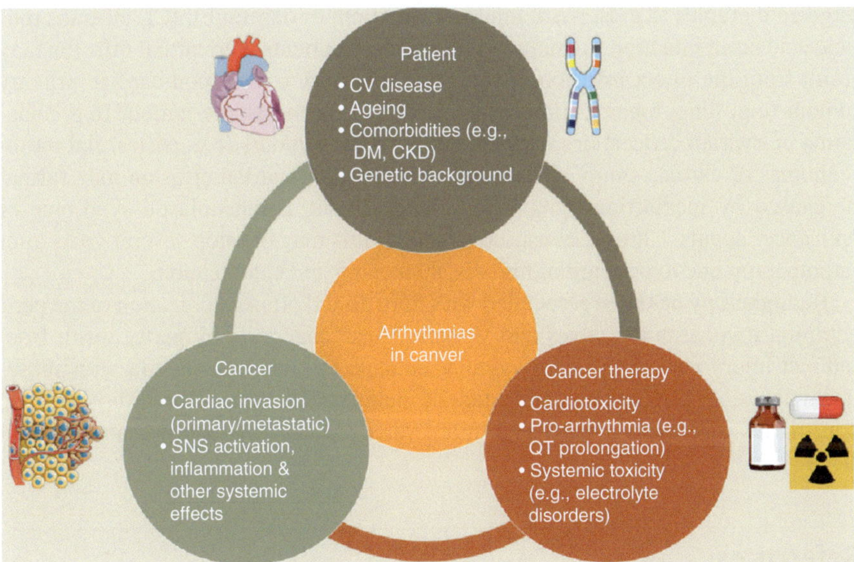

Fig. 4.5 Pathophysiology of arrhythmias in patients with cancer. (Reprinted with permission from Farmakis and Filippatos [3])

patient-related factors may also predispose to arrhythmias. These factors include ageing, which is a common risk factor for CV disease and cancer and is associated with specific rhythm disturbances such as atrial fibrillation or sick sinus syndrome; concomitant CV disease; non-CV comorbidities, such as diabetes mellitus or chronic kidney disease; and genetic factors, such as inherited QT prolongation [3].

Two typical forms of rhythm disturbances seen in cancer patients and potentially related to anticancer therapy are QT prolongation and atrial fibrillation (AFib). Many cancer drugs, particularly arsenic trioxide and TKI, such as vandetanib and lapatinib, may cause QT prolongation, which may further be accentuated by other QT-prolonging medications that the patient might receive in parallel, electrolyte disturbances caused by cancer or its therapy and pre-existing/inherited QT prolongation [1]. On the other hand, cancer and atrial fibrillation share many common risk factors that predispose to both conditions, while certain anticancer drugs, such as the Bruton tyrosine kinase inhibitor ibrutinib, and mainly cancer surgery, particularly lung resection, may induce atrial fibrillation [6].

Pericardial and Valvular Disease

Pericardial disease in cancer patients may include acute pericarditis, pericardial effusion, often complicated by tamponade, and chronic constrictive pericarditis. Acute pericarditis can be caused by chest irradiation (e.g. for lung or oesophageal cancer), chemotherapy (e.g. anthracyclines, bleomycin, cyclophosphamide), targeted therapies (e.g. Bcr-Abl inhibitors imatinib or dasatinib), ICI, all-trans retinoic acid or an infection in immunocompromised patients. Pericardial effusion may result from the direct invasion of the pericardium by a local non-cardiac primary tumour (e.g. lung, breast, or oesophageal cancer), a metastatic tumour (e.g. melanoma or ovarian cancer) or rarely primary cardiac tumours (e.g. pericardial mesotheliomas or cardiac synovial sarcomas) [52, 53]. Pericardial effusion may further be caused by mediastinal lymph node involvement, paraneoplastic syndrome or anticancer agents. Chronic constrictive pericarditis may develop several years after radiotherapy due to pericardial fibrosis, thickening and calcification.

Radiotherapy has been associated with fibrosis and often calcification of the pericardium, myocardium, valves and vessels. These changes may partly result from indirect injury caused by microvascular damage that led to ischemia with subsequent fibrosis [12]. Clinical manifestations include acute peri−/myocarditis, chronic constrictive pericarditis, aortic and mitral valve calcification and late aortic stenosis [44].

References

1. Zamorano JL, Lancellotti P, Rodriguez Muñoz D, Aboyans V, Asteggiano R, Galderisi M, Habib G, Lenihan DJ, Lip GYH, Lyon AR, Lopez Fernandez T, Mohty D, Piepoli MF, Tamargo J, Torbicki A, Suter TM, Zamorano JL, Aboyans V, Achenbach S, Agewall S, Badimon L, Barón-Esquivias G, Baumgartner H, Bax JJ, Bueno H, Carerj S, Dean V, Erol Ç, Fitzsimons D, Gaemperli O, et al. 2016 ESC position paper on cancer treatments and cardiovascular toxicity developed under the auspices of the ESC committee for practice guidelines: the task Force for cancer treatments and cardiovascular toxicity of the European Society of Cardiology (ESC). Eur J Heart Fail. 2017;19:9–42.
2. Farmakis D, Mantzourani M, Filippatos G. Anthracycline-induced cardiomyopathy: secrets and lies. Eur J Heart Fail. 2018;20:907–9.
3. Farmakis D, Filippatos G. Arrhythmias in cancer: rhythm is gonna get you! Eur J Heart Fail. 2021;23:154–6.
4. Farmakis D, Keramida K, Filippatos G. How to build a cardio-oncology service? Eur J Heart Fail. 2018;20:1732–4.
5. Lyon AR, Dent S, Stanway S, Earl H, Brezden-Masley C, Cohen-Solal A, Tocchetti CG, Moslehi JJ, Groarke JD, Bergler-Klein J, Khoo V, Tan LL, Anker MS, von Haehling S, Maack C, Pudil R, Barac A, Thavendiranathan P, Ky B, Neilan TG, Belenkov Y, Rosen SD, Iakobishvili Z, Sverdlov AL, Hajjar LA, AVS M, Manisty C, Ciardiello F, Farmakis D, de Boer RA, et al. Baseline cardiovascular risk assessment in cancer patients scheduled to receive cardiotoxic cancer therapies: a position statement and new risk assessment tools from the Cardio-Oncology Study Group of the Heart Failure Association of the European Society of Cardiology in collaboration with the International Cardio-Oncology Society. Eur J Heart Fail. 2020;22:1945–60.
6. Farmakis D, Parissis J, Filippatos G. Insights into onco-cardiology: atrial fibrillation in cancer. J Am Coll Cardiol. 2014;63:945–53.
7. de Boer RA, Hulot J-S, Tocchetti CG, Aboumsallem JP, Ameri P, Anker SD, Bauersachs J, Bertero E, AJS C, Čelutkienė J, Chioncel O, Dodion P, Eschenhagen T, Farmakis D, Bayes-Genis A, Jäger D, Jankowska EA, Kitsis RN, Konety SH, Larkin J, Lehmann L, Lenihan DJ, Maack C, Moslehi JJ, Müller OJ, Nowak-Sliwinska P, Piepoli MF, Ponikowski P, Pudil R, Rainer PP, et al. Common mechanistic pathways in cancer and heart failure. A scientific roadmap on behalf of the Translational Research Committee of the Heart Failure Association (HFA) of the European Society of Cardiology (ESC). Eur J Heart Fail. 2020;22:2272–89.

8. Čelutkienė J, Pudil R, López-Fernández T, Grapsa J, Nihoyannopoulos P, Bergler-Klein J, Cohen-Solal A, Farmakis D, Tocchetti CG, von Haehling S, Barberis V, Flachskampf FA, Čeponienė I, Haegler-Laube E, Suter T, Lapinskas T, Prasad S, de Boer RA, Wechalekar K, Anker MS, Iakobishvili Z, Bucciarelli-Ducci C, Schulz-Menger J, Cosyns B, Gaemperli O, Belenkov Y, Hulot J-S, Galderisi M, Lancellotti P, Bax J, et al. Role of cardiovascular imaging in cancer patients receiving cardiotoxic therapies: a position statement on behalf of the Heart Failure Association (HFA), the European Association of Cardiovascular Imaging (EACVI) and the Cardio-Oncology Council of the European Society of Cardiology (ESC). Eur J Heart Fail. 2020;22:1504–24.

9. Pudil R, Mueller C, Čelutkienė J, Henriksen PA, Lenihan D, Dent S, Barac A, Stanway S, Moslehi J, Suter TM, Ky B, Štěrba M, Cardinale D, Cohen-Solal A, Tocchetti CG, Farmakis D, Bergler-Klein J, Anker MS, Von Haehling S, Belenkov Y, Iakobishvili Z, Maack C, Ciardiello F, Ruschitzka F, AJS C, Seferovic P, Lainscak M, Piepoli MF, Chioncel O, Bax J, et al. Role of serum biomarkers in cancer patients receiving cardiotoxic cancer therapies: a position statement from the Cardio-Oncology Study Group of the Heart Failure Association and the Cardio-Oncology Council of the European Society of Cardiology. Eur J Heart Fail. 2020;22:1966–83.

10. Suter TM, Ewer MS. Cancer drugs and the heart: importance and management. Eur Heart J. 2013;34:1102–11.

11. Ewer MS, Ewer SM. Cardiotoxicity of anticancer treatments. Nat Rev Cardiol. 2015;12:547–58.

12. Lenneman CG, Sawyer DB. Cardio-oncology: an update on cardiotoxicity of cancer-related treatment. Circ Res. 2016;118:1008–20.

13. Vejpongsa P, Yeh ETH. Prevention of anthracycline-induced cardiotoxicity: challenges and opportunities. J Am Coll Cardiol. 2014;64:938–45.

14. Postow MA, Callahan MK, Wolchok JD. Immune checkpoint blockade in cancer therapy. J Clin Oncol Off J Am Soc Clin Oncol. 2015;33:1974–82.

15. Puzanov I, Diab A, Abdallah K, Bingham CO, Brogdon C, Dadu R, Hamad L, Kim S, Lacouture ME, NR LB, Lenihan D, Onofrei C, Shannon V, Sharma R, Silk AW, Skondra D, Suarez-Almazor ME, Wang Y, Wiley K, Kaufman HL, Ernstoff MS, Society for Immunotherapy of Cancer Toxicity Management Working Group. Managing toxicities associated with immune checkpoint inhibitors: consensus recommendations from the Society for Immunotherapy of Cancer (SITC) Toxicity Management Working Group. J Immunother Cancer. 2017;5:95.

16. Hu J-R, Florido R, Lipson EJ, Naidoo J, Ardehali R, Tocchetti CG, Lyon AR, Padera RF, Johnson DB, Moslehi J. Cardiovascular toxicities associated with immune checkpoint inhibitors. Cardiovasc Res. 2019;115:854–68.

17. Mahmood SS, Fradley MG, Cohen JV, Nohria A, Reynolds KL, Heinzerling LM, Sullivan RJ, Damrongwatanasuk R, Chen CL, Gupta D, Kirchberger MC, Awadalla M, Hassan MZO, Moslehi JJ, Shah SP, Ganatra S, Thavendiranathan P, Lawrence DP, Groarke JD, Neilan TG. Myocarditis in patients treated with immune checkpoint inhibitors. J Am Coll Cardiol. 2018;71:1755–64.

18. Salem J-E, Manouchehri A, Moey M, Lebrun-Vignes B, Bastarache L, Pariente A, Gobert A, Spano J-P, Balko JM, Bonaca MP, Roden DM, Johnson DB, Moslehi JJ. Cardiovascular toxicities associated with immune checkpoint inhibitors: an observational, retrospective, pharmacovigilance study. Lancet Oncol. 2018;19:1579–89.

19. Stangl K, Stangl V. The ubiquitin-proteasome pathway and endothelial (dys)function. Cardiovasc Res. 2010;85:281–90.

20. Dimopoulos MA, Moreau P, Palumbo A, Joshua D, Pour L, Hájek R, Facon T, Ludwig H, Oriol A, Goldschmidt H, Rosiñol L, Straub J, Suvorov A, Araujo C, Rimashevskaya E, Pika T, Gaidano G, Weisel K, Goranova-Marinova V, Schwarer A, Minuk L, Masszi T, Karamanesht I, Offidani M, Hungria V, Spencer A, Orlowski RZ, Gillenwater HH, Mohamed N, Feng S, et al. Carfilzomib and dexamethasone versus bortezomib and dexamethasone for patients with relapsed or refractory multiple myeloma (ENDEAVOR): a randomised, phase 3, open-label, multicentre study. Lancet Oncol. 2016;17:27–38.

21. Stewart AK, Rajkumar SV, Dimopoulos MA, Masszi T, Špička I, Oriol A, Hájek R, Rosiñol L, Siegel DS, Mihaylov GG, Goranova-Marinova V, Rajnics P, Suvorov A, Niesvizky R,

Jakubowiak AJ, San-Miguel JF, Ludwig H, Wang M, Maisnar V, Minarik J, Bensinger WI, Mateos M-V, Ben-Yehuda D, Kukreti V, Zojwalla N, Tonda ME, Yang X, Xing B, Moreau P, Palumbo A, et al. Carfilzomib, lenalidomide, and dexamethasone for relapsed multiple myeloma. N Engl J Med. 2015;372:142–52.

22. Shah C, Bishnoi R, Jain A, Bejjanki H, Xiong S, Wang Y, Zou F, Moreb JS. Cardiotoxicity associated with carfilzomib: systematic review and meta-analysis. Leuk Lymphoma. 2018;59:2557–69.

23. Long GV, Stroyakovskiy D, Gogas H, Levchenko E, de Braud F, Larkin J, Garbe C, Jouary T, Hauschild A, Grob J-J, Chiarion-Sileni V, Lebbe C, Mandalà M, Millward M, Arance A, Bondarenko I, JBAG H, Hansson J, Utikal J, Ferraresi V, Kovalenko N, Mohr P, Probachai V, Schadendorf D, Nathan P, Robert C, Ribas A, DJ DM, Irani JG, Swann S, et al. Dabrafenib and trametinib versus dabrafenib and placebo for Val600 BRAF-mutant melanoma: a multicentre, double-blind, phase 3 randomised controlled trial. Lancet Lond Engl. 2015;386:444–51.

24. Marber MS, Rose B, Wang Y. The p38 mitogen-activated protein kinase pathway--a potential target for intervention in infarction, hypertrophy, and heart failure. J Mol Cell Cardiol. 2011;51:485–90.

25. Hu LA, Chen W, Martin NP, Whalen EJ, Premont RT, Lefkowitz RJ. GIPC interacts with the beta1-adrenergic receptor and regulates beta1-adrenergic receptor-mediated ERK activation. J Biol Chem. 2003;278:26295–301.

26. Herrmann J, Yang EH, Iliescu CA, Cilingiroglu M, Charitakis K, Hakeem A, Toutouzas K, Leesar MA, Grines CL, Marmagkiolis K. Vascular toxicities of cancer therapies: the old and the new–an evolving avenue. Circulation. 2016;133:1272–89.

27. Karaman S, Leppänen VM, Alitalo K. Vascular endothelial growth factor signaling in development and disease. Development. 2018;145(14):dev151019.

28. Campia U, Moslehi JJ, Amiri-Kordestani L, Barac A, Beckman JA, Chism DD, Cohen P, Groarke JD, Herrmann J, Reilly CM, Weintraub NL. Cardio-oncology: vascular and metabolic perspectives: a scientific statement from the American Heart Association. Circulation. 2019;139:e579–602.

29. De Keulenaer GW, Feyen E, Dugaucquier L, Shakeri H, Shchendrygina A, Belenkov YN, Brink M, Vermeulen Z, Segers VFM. Mechanisms of the multitasking endothelial protein NRG-1 as a compensatory factor during chronic heart failure. Circ Heart Fail. 2019;12:e006288.

30. van Dijk CG, Nieuweboer FE, Pei JY, Xu YJ, Burgisser P, van Mulligen E, el Azzouzi H, Duncker DJ, Verhaar MC. The complex mural cell: pericyte function in health and disease. Int J Cardiol. 2015;190:75–89.

31. Chintalgattu V, Rees ML, Culver JC, Goel A, Jiffar T, Zhang J, Jr KD, Pati S, Bankson JA, Pasqualini R, Arap W, Bryan NS, Taegtmeyer H, Langley RR, Yao H, Kupferman ME, Entman ML, Dickinson ME, Khakoo AY. Coronary microvascular pericytes are the cellular target of sunitinib malate-induced cardiotoxicity. Sci Transl Med. 2013;5(187):187ra69.

32. Neves KB, Rios FJ, Jones R, Evans TRJ, Montezano AC, Touyz RM. Microparticles from vascular endothelial growth factor pathway inhibitor-treated cancer patients mediate endothelial cell injury. Cardiovasc Res. 2019;115:978–88.

33. Ferrara N. VEGF-A: a critical regulator of blood vessel growth. Eur Cytokine Netw. 2009;20:158–63.

34. Scappaticci FA, Skillings JR, Holden SN, Gerber H-P, Miller K, Kabbinavar F, Bergsland E, Ngai J, Holmgren E, Wang J, Hurwitz H. Arterial thromboembolic events in patients with metastatic carcinoma treated with chemotherapy and bevacizumab. J Natl Cancer Inst. 2007;99:1232–9.

35. Chu TF, Rupnick MA, Kerkela R, Dallabrida SM, Zurakowski D, Nguyen L, Woulfe K, Pravda E, Cassiola F, Desai J, George S, Morgan JA, Harris DM, Ismail NS, Chen J-H, Schoen FJ, Van den Abbeele AD, Demetri GD, Force T, Chen MH. Cardiotoxicity associated with tyrosine kinase inhibitor sunitinib. Lancet Lond Engl. 2007;370:2011–9.

36. Khakoo AY, Kassiotis CM, Tannir N, Plana JC, Halushka M, Bickford C, Trent J, Champion JC, Durand J-B, Lenihan DJ. Heart failure associated with sunitinib malate: a multitargeted receptor tyrosine kinase inhibitor. Cancer. 2008;112:2500–8.

37. Chislock EM, Ring C, Pendergast AM. Abl kinases are required for vascular function, Tie2 expression, and angiopoietin-1-mediated survival. Proc Natl Acad Sci U S A. 2013;110:12432–7.
38. Kerkelä R, Grazette L, Yacobi R, Iliescu C, Patten R, Beahm C, Walters B, Shevtsov S, Pesant S, Clubb FJ, Rosenzweig A, Salomon RN, Van Etten RA, Alroy J, Durand JB, Force T. Cardiotoxicity of the cancer therapeutic agent imatinib mesylate. Nat Med. 2006;12:908–16.
39. Douxfils J, Haguet H, Mullier F, Chatelain C, Graux C, Dogné J-M. Association between BCR-ABL tyrosine kinase inhibitors for chronic myeloid leukemia and cardiovascular events, major molecular response, and overall survival: a systematic review and meta-analysis. JAMA Oncol. 2016;2:625–32.
40. Polk A, Vistisen K, Vaage-Nilsen M, Nielsen DL. A systematic review of the pathophysiology of 5-fluorouracil-induced cardiotoxicity. BMC Pharmacol Toxicol. 2014;15:47.
41. Jafri M, Protheroe A. Cisplatin-associated thrombosis. Anti-Cancer Drugs. 2008;19:927–9.
42. Nuver J, De Haas EC, Van Zweeden M, Gietema JA, Meijer C. Vascular damage in testicular cancer patients: a study on endothelial activation by bleomycin and cisplatin in vitro. Oncol Rep. 2010;23:247–53.
43. Brouwers EEM, Huitema ADR, Beijnen JH, Schellens JHM. Long-term platinum retention after treatment with cisplatin and oxaliplatin. BMC Clin Pharmacol. 2008;8:7.
44. Groarke JD, Nguyen PL, Nohria A, Ferrari R, Cheng S, Moslehi J. Cardiovascular complications of radiation therapy for thoracic malignancies: the role for non-invasive imaging for detection of cardiovascular disease. Eur Heart J. 2014;35:612–23.
45. Venkatesulu BP, Mahadevan LS, Aliru ML, Yang X, Bodd MH, Singh PK, Yusuf SW, Abe JI, Krishnan S. Radiation-induced endothelial vascular injury: a review of possible mechanisms. JACC Basic Transl Sci. 2018;3:563–72.
46. Vatanen A, Sarkola T, Ojala TH, Turanlahti M, Jahnukainen T, Saarinen-Pihkala UM, Jahnukainen K. Radiotherapy-related arterial intima thickening and plaque formation in childhood cancer survivors detected with very-high resolution ultrasound during young adulthood. Pediatr Blood Cancer. 2015;62:2000–6.
47. Khorana AA, Francis CW, Culakova E, Kuderer NM, Lyman GH. Thromboembolism is a leading cause of death in cancer patients receiving outpatient chemotherapy. J Thromb Haemost JTH. 2007;5:632–4.
48. Donnellan E, Khorana AA. Cancer and venous thromboembolic disease: a review. Oncologist. 2017;22:199–207.
49. Ay C, Pabinger I, Cohen AT. Cancer-associated venous thromboembolism: burden, mechanisms, and management. Thromb Haemost. 2017;117:219–30.
50. Mosarla RC, Vaduganathan M, Qamar A, Moslehi J, Piazza G, Giugliano RP. Anticoagulation strategies in patients with cancer: JACC review topic of the week. J Am Coll Cardiol. 2019;73:1336–49.
51. Tisdale JE, Chung MK, Campbell KB, Hammadah M, Joglar JA, Leclerc J, Rajagopalan B, American Heart Association Clinical Pharmacology Committee of the Council on Clinical Cardiology and Council on Cardiovascular and Stroke Nursing. Drug-induced arrhythmias: a scientific statement from the American Heart Association. Circulation. 2020;142:e214–33.
52. Burazor I, Imazio M, Markel G, Adler Y. Malignant pericardial effusion. Cardiology. 2013;124:224–32.
53. Sánchez-Enrique C, Nuñez-Gil IJ, Viana-Tejedor A, De Agustín A, Vivas D, Palacios-Rubio J, Vilchez JP, Cecconi A, Macaya C, Fernández-Ortiz A. Cause and long-term outcome of cardiac tamponade. Am J Cardiol. 2016;117:664–9.

Cardiac Risk Factors for Immunotherapy

5

Andreina Carbone, Vincenzo Quagliariello, Martina Iovine,
Maria Laura Canale, and Nicola Maurea

Although immunotherapy has significantly improved the outcome of many types of cancer, it is associated with adverse events, mainly gastrointestinal and endocrine immune effects, and to a lesser extent, cardiotoxicity, which is usually serious and associated with a high mortality [1]. Cardiotoxicity is defined as any heart injury (functional or structural) due to disease treatment. Data about cardiotoxicity related to immunotherapy is increasing as this treatment becomes more widespread. Immunotherapy-related cardiotoxicity affects 0.9–3.17% of all cancer patients [2–4]. Escudier et al. [5] reported that among patients who developed cardiotoxicity, one-third of the deaths were caused by cardiological injury. Notably, the most common manifestations of cardiac toxicity are myocarditis, which occurs in 0.5–2% of individuals treated with checkpoint inhibitors and is associated with major adverse cardiac events in 50% of cases [3, 5], pericardial disease (pericarditis, pericardial effusion, and cardiac tamponade), conduction disorders and arrhythmias (atrial fibrillation, ventricular arrhythmias, Takotsubo cardiomyopathy) [5]. Therefore, given the above, all patients treated with immunotherapy should advise their physician if they experience dyspnea, palpitations, dizziness, chest pain, or syncope, because such symptoms could be related to cardiotoxicity. In case these manifestations occur, patients should undergo a careful diagnostic workup.

It is not yet possible to identify patients at high or low risk of immune checkpoint-induced cardiotoxicity since serious adverse events can occur in both heart patients and patients without cardiovascular disease. Cardiotoxicity may develop in the

A. Carbone · V. Quagliariello · M. Iovine
National Cancer Institute, IRCCS Pascale, Naples, Italy
e-mail: v.quagliariello@istitutotumori.na.it; martina.iovine@istitutotumori.na.it

M. L. Canale
Cardiology, Versilia Hospital, Azienda USL Toscana Nord Ovest - Lido di Camaiore (LU), Toscana, Italy

N. Maurea (✉)
Istituto Nazionale Tumori IRCCS Fondazione G. Pascale, Napoli, Italy
e-mail: n.maurea@istitutotumori.na.it

A. Russo et al. (eds.), *Cardio-Oncology*, Current Clinical Pathology, https://doi.org/10.1007/978-3-030-97744-3_5

absence of a history of significant cardiac risk factors and may be associated with more general myositis [2]. In pharmacovigilance studies, the incidence of myocarditis was higher in patients treated with the combination of nivolumab plus ipilimumab than in patients receiving nivolumab alone (0.27% versus 0.06%), which suggests that combination therapy might be a factor for cardiovascular toxicity [6]. In an observational study, Mahmood et al. [3] showed that the possible risk factors for immunotherapy-related cardiotoxicity are previous heart disease (past myocardial infarction and heart failure), previous anthracycline treatment, a history of drug-related cardiomyopathy (disease of the heart muscle), the coexistence of autoimmune diseases (systemic lupus erythematosus, Sjogren's syndrome, and sarcoidosis), and concomitant use of another type of oncological treatment (e.g., vascular endothelial growth factor and tyrosine kinase inhibitors) [3]. In the same study, they also showed that an increased risk of cardiotoxicity related to immunotherapy can occur in patients with diabetes, sleep apnea, and an elevated body mass index [3]. Furthermore, they found that a previous reduced left ventricular ejection fraction did not appear to impact on cardiotoxicity incidence and prognosis: indeed, 38% of major adverse cardiovascular events occurred in patients with preserved ejection fraction [3]. Lastly, it remains to be established whether or not global longitudinal strain assessment can identify patients at high risk of cardiotoxicity.

Apart from risk factors, all patients should undergo a thorough cardiac evaluation before starting immunotherapy. The aim of a baseline evaluation is to recognize subjects who have an underlying cardiac condition or cardiovascular risk factors and could thus be at risk of drug-related adverse events. Furthermore, the most severe modifiable cardiovascular risk factors (diabetes, hypertension, obesity, and smoking) should be treated and patients stratified into low, moderate, high, and very high risk according to international guidelines [7–9], in order to minimize the conditions that might synergize with the cardiotoxic effect of immunotherapy and result in a worse prognosis. Table 5.1 summarizes the potential cardiac and noncardiac risk factors for immunotherapy-related cardiotoxicity.

Table 5.1 Cardiac and noncardiac risk factors for immunotherapy-related cardiotoxicity

Cardiac risk factors
Previous heart disease (myocardial infarction, heart failure)
History of drug-related cardiomyopathy
Diabetes mellitus, arterial hypertension, dyslipidemia, smoking, obesity
Sleep apnea syndrome
Noncardiac risk factors
Previous anthracycline treatment
Concomitant use of another type of oncological treatment (e.g., vascular endothelial growth factor and tyrosine kinase inhibitors)
Autoimmune disease (systemic lupus erythematosus, Sjogren's syndrome, sarcoidosis)

Why Evaluate the Cardiovascular Risk in Oncological Patients Who Have Undergone Immunotherapy?

Cardiovascular disease and cancer are the two main causes of death worldwide and share many risk factors, namely, smoking, obesity, sedentary lifestyle, an "unhealthy" diet (rich in animal fats and low in vegetables and fiber), alcohol abuse, diabetes, and metabolic syndrome [10]. Notwithstanding the treatment-related improvement in life expectancy of cancer patients recorded in recent decades, treatment can have negative effects and often exacerbate the cardiovascular risk profile [10], thereby increasing the risk of cardiovascular events in people who have recovered from cancer. A high cardiovascular risk complicates the management of cancer patients: it amplifies the risk of cardiovascular events following cancer immunotherapies and limits therapeutic options. Lastly, such cardiac risk factors as obesity, diabetes, and cigarette smoking also have a negative impact on cancer treatment and prognosis.

How to Quantify Cardiovascular Risk?

Patients at a high cardiovascular risk or with structural heart disease are usually excluded from randomized clinical trials (RCTs) that test cancer therapies. Therefore, data from RCTs and meta-analyses may not be reliable in the cardio-oncology setting. Consequently, score systems have been devised to evaluate the risk of cardiovascular events. The European Society of Cardiology classifies patients into four classes of increasing cardiovascular risk (low, moderate, high, and very high risk) (Table 5.2) based on the presence/absence of heart disease or of diseases that have a strong impact on the cardiovascular system (e.g., diabetes) or on a cardiovascular risk factor score [7–9]. Once a patient's cardiovascular risk is identified, their therapeutic program and the intensity of patient care and monitoring can be established. Regarding the objectives of treatment, in the absence of cardio-oncology and immunotherapy data, cardiovascular risk can be evaluated according to the guidelines of the relevant scientific societies [7–9].

Experimental Preventive Strategies for Immune Checkpoint Inhibitor (ICI)-Induced Cardiotoxicity: Evidence and Perspectives

The mechanisms underlying cardiac toxicity have yet to be clarified. Khunger et al. [11] reported that ICI-induced cardiotoxicity results from uncontrolled lymphocyte infiltration into the myocardium and the consequent induction of cell necrosis and apoptosis. However, based on the direct and indirect interactions between lymphocytes and cardiac cells, several strategies aimed at decreasing the cross-reactivity and production of pro-inflammatory and pro-fibrotic cytokines are currently under study [12, 13]. Firstly, treatment with glucocorticoids was found to improve left ventricular function in ICI-treated patients and could therefore be used to prevent

Table 5.2 Cardiovascular risk assessment according to the European Society of Cardiology guidelines [8]

Very high risk	Documented atherosclerotic cardiovascular disease (previous acute coronary syndrome, stable angina, coronary revascularization, stroke and transient ischemic attack, and peripheral arterial disease). Also includes significant plaque on coronary angiography or CT scan (multivessel coronary disease with two major epicardial arteries having >50% stenosis) or on carotid ultrasound Diabetes mellitus with target organ damage, or at least three major risk factors, or early onset of type 1 diabetes of long duration (>20 years) Severe chronic kidney disease (eGFR <30 mL/min/1.73 m^2) A calculated SCORE of ≥10% for 10-year risk of fatal cardiovascular disease Familiar hyperlipidemia with atherosclerotic cardiovascular disease or with another major risk factor
High risk	Markedly elevated single risk factors: triglycerides >8 mmol/L (>310 mg/dL), LDL-cholesterol >4.9 mmol/L (>190 mg/dL), or blood pressure ≥ 180/110 mmHg Patients with familiar hyperlipidemia without other major risk factors Patients with diabetes mellitus without target organ damage, with duration ≥10 years or another additional risk factor Moderate chronic kidney disease (eGFR 30–59 mL/min/1.73 m^2) A calculated SCORE ≥ 5% and < 10% for 10-year risk of fatal cardiovascular disease
Moderate risk	Young patients (type 1 diabetes <35 years; type 2 diabetes <50 years) with duration <10 years, without other risk factors Calculated SCORE of ≥1% and < 5% for 10-year risk of fatal cardiovascular disease
Low risk	Calculated SCORE of <1% for 10-year risk of fatal cardiovascular disease

SCORE, Systematic Coronary Risk Estimation; eGFR, estimated glomerular filtration rate. The electronic version of SCORE, HeartScore (http://www.heartscore.org/en_GB/)

ICI-induced cardiotoxicity [14]. The main mechanism of glucocorticoid-related cardioprotective effects during treatment with ICI is through inhibiting the accumulation of lymphocytes (T cells, B cells, and NK cells), monocytes, and dendritic cells in cardiac tissue [14]; the reduced myocardial lymphocyte infiltration determines the reduction of cardiac fibrosis and myocarditis in these patients [14]. Various other treatment regimens have been proposed, ranging from 30 mg of oral prednisone daily for isolated pericardial disease to 1000 mg of intravenous methylprednisolone daily for fulminant myocardial disease [15, 16]. A strategy currently used in clinical practice to treat patients without fulminant myocarditis is the oral administration of prednisone at 1–2 mg/kg daily followed by a slow taper [17, 18]. Other immunosuppressive regimens used to treat steroid nonresponders are plasmapheresis [19], intravenous immunoglobulins [20], anti-thymocyte globulin [21], mycophenolate mofetil [22], tacrolimus [23], and infliximab [24]. However, data supporting their use are lacking, which limits their use in the treatment of cardiac toxicities.

Another promising experimental strategy is abatacept, a CTLA-4 analogue that reduces ipilimumab-induced cardiotoxicity [25]. In preclinical studies, in mice treated with ICI, the administration of abatacept decreased the incidence of myocarditis and normalized serum markers of cardiovascular injuries [26]. A patient treated with a CTLA-4 blocking agent experienced a refractory syndrome to glucocorticoids; in an attempt to reduce the incidence of myocarditis, intravenous abatacept was administered at a dose of 500 mg every 2 weeks for a total of five doses. Abatacept rapidly decreased troponin levels and symptoms of myocarditis (arrhythmias) and myositis (muscular weakness and facial paralysis) [25].

Lastly, there is an urgent need to develop clinical guidelines for the early diagnosis and treatment of ICI-induced cardiotoxicity. Currently, there are no treatment guidelines for these potentially fatal side effects, and high-dose steroids remain the cornerstone of therapy, as with immune-related adverse events in any organ system. Clinical studies to find an effective cardioprotective agent for ICI-treated cancer patients remain a hot topic in cardio-oncology.

References

1. Jagielska B, Ozdowska P, Gepner K, Kubala S, Siedlecki JA, Sarnowski TJ, et al. Cardiotoxicity danger in immunotherapy. IUBMB Life. 2020;72(6):1160–7.
2. Zimmer L, Goldinger SM, Hofmann L, Loquai C, Ugurel S, Thomas I, et al. Neurological, respiratory, musculoskeletal, cardiac and ocular side-effects of anti-PD-1 therapy. Eur J Cancer. 2016;60:210–25.
3. Mahmood SS, Fradley MG, Cohen JV, Nohria A, Reynolds KL, Heinzerling LM, et al. Myocarditis in patients treated with immune checkpoint inhibitors. J Am Coll Cardiol. 2018;71(16):1755–64.
4. Asnani A. Cardiotoxicity of immunotherapy: incidence, diagnosis, and management. Curr Oncol Rep. 2018;20(6):44.
5. Escudier M, Cautela J, Malissen N, Ancedy Y, Orabona M, Pinto J, et al. Clinical features, management, and outcomes of immune checkpoint inhibitor-related cardiotoxicity. Circulation. 2017;136(21):2085–7.
6. Johnson DB, Balko JM, Compton ML, Chalkias S, Gorham J, Xu Y, et al. Fulminant myocarditis with combination immune checkpoint blockade. N Engl J Med. 2016;375(18):1749–55.
7. Mach F, Baigent C, Catapano AL, Koskinas KC, Casula M, Badimon L, et al. 2019 ESC/EAS guidelines for the management of dyslipidaemias: lipid modification to reduce cardiovascular risk. Eur Heart J. 2020;41(1):111–88.
8. Williams B, Mancia G, Spiering W, Agabiti Rosei E, Azizi M, Burnier M, et al. 2018 ESC/ESH guidelines for the management of arterial hypertension. Eur Heart J. 2018;39(33):3021–104.
9. Piepoli MF, Hoes AW, Agewall S, Albus C, Brotons C, Catapano AL, et al. 2016 European Guidelines on cardiovascular disease prevention in clinical practice: The Sixth Joint Task Force of the European Society of Cardiology and Other Societies on Cardiovascular Disease Prevention in Clinical Practice (constituted by representatives of 10 societies and by invited experts) Developed with the special contribution of the European Association for Cardiovascular Prevention & Rehabilitation (EACPR). Eur Heart J. 2016;37(29):2315–81.
10. de Haas EC, Oosting SF, Lefrandt JD, Wolffenbuttel BH, Sleijfer DT, Gietema JA. The metabolic syndrome in cancer survivors. Lancet Oncol. 2010;11(2):193–203.
11. Khunger A, Battel L, Wadhawan A, More A, Kapoor A, Agrawal N. New insights into mechanisms of immune checkpoint inhibitor-induced cardiovascular toxicity. Curr Oncol Rep. 2020;22(7):65.
12. Quagliariello V, Passariello M, Coppola C, Rea D, Barbieri A, Scherillo M, et al. Cardiotoxicity and pro-inflammatory effects of the immune checkpoint inhibitor Pembrolizumab associated to Trastuzumab. Int J Cardiol. 2019;292:171–9.
13. Varricchi G, Galdiero MR, Marone G, Criscuolo G, Triassi M, Bonaduce D, et al. Cardiotoxicity of immune checkpoint inhibitors. ESMO Open. 2017;2(4):e000247.

14. Michel L, Rassaf T, Totzeck M. Cardiotoxicity from immune checkpoint inhibitors. Int J Cardiol Heart Vasc. 2019;25:100420.
15. Nakashima H, Umeyama Y, Minami K. Successive immunosuppressive treatment of fulminant myocarditis that is refractory to mechanical circulatory support. Am J Case Rep. 2013;14:116–9.
16. Veronese G, Ammirati E, Cipriani M, Frigerio M. Fulminant myocarditis: characteristics, treatment, and outcomes. Anatol J Cardiol. 2018;19(4):279–86.
17. Rudzki JD. Management of adverse events related to checkpoint inhibition therapy. Memo. 2018;11(2):132–7.
18. Williams KJ, Grauer DW, Henry DW, Rockey ML. Corticosteroids for the management of immune-related adverse events in patients receiving checkpoint inhibitors. J Oncol Pharm Pract. 2019;25(3):544–50.
19. Psimaras D, Velasco R, Birzu C, Tamburin S, Lustberg M, Bruna J, et al. Immune checkpoint inhibitors-induced neuromuscular toxicity: from pathogenesis to treatment. J Peripheral Nerv Syst. 2019;24(Suppl 2):S74–85.
20. Kim A, Keam B, Cheun H, Lee ST, Gook HS, Han MK. Immune-checkpoint-inhibitor-induced severe autoimmune encephalitis treated by steroid and intravenous immunoglobulin. J Clin Neurol. 2019;15(2):259–61.
21. Jain V, Mohebtash M, Rodrigo ME, Ruiz G, Atkins MB, Barac A. Autoimmune myocarditis caused by immune checkpoint inhibitors treated with antithymocyte globulin. J Immunother. 2018;41(7):332–5.
22. Mir R, Shaw HM, Nathan PD. Mycophenolate mofetil alongside high-dose corticosteroids: optimizing the management of combination immune checkpoint inhibitor-induced colitis. Melanoma Res. 2019;29(1):102–6.
23. Beardslee T, Draper A, Kudchadkar R. Tacrolimus for the treatment of immune-related adverse effects refractory to systemic steroids and anti-tumor necrosis factor alpha therapy. J Oncol Pharm Pract. 2019;25(5):1275–81.
24. Agrawal N, Khunger A, Vachhani P, Colvin TA, Hattoum A, Spangenthal E, et al. Cardiac toxicity associated with immune checkpoint inhibitors: case series and review of the literature. Case Rep Oncol. 2019;12(1):260–76.
25. Choi J, Lee SY. Clinical characteristics and treatment of immune-related adverse events of immune checkpoint inhibitors. Immune Network. 2020;20(1):e9.
26. Salem JE, Allenbach Y, Vozy A, Brechot N, Johnson DB, Moslehi JJ, et al. Abatacept for severe immune checkpoint inhibitor-associated myocarditis. N Engl J Med. 2019;380(24):2377–9.

Diagnostic Methods of Cardiac Immunotherapy Damaging

6

Girolamo Manno, Daniela Di Lisi, and Giuseppina Novo

Introduction

In the last years, the survival of cancer patients has definitely improved, thanks to the advances in early diagnosis, staging, and therapy [1]. But at the same time, this caused an increasing burden of complications related to cancer treatment. Among these, the main ones are represented by cardiovascular complications [2]. Therefore, a new branch of cardiology is born, named "cardio-oncology" with the aim of preventing cardiovascular complications related to antineoplastic treatment, early diagnosis, and treatment of any complications and allowing the completion of the expected antineoplastic treatment [2–4]. Although clinical evaluation is always the cornerstone for overall patient approach, when symptoms arise clearly, cardiovascular damage is already advanced; therefore, it is recommended, after a baseline evaluation, to monitor cardiac function to promptly detect any variation [3, 5]. Many strategies are available to monitor cardiac function during or after chemotherapy including cardiac imaging (echocardiography, magnetic resonance, nuclear imaging) and laboratory markers (troponin, natriuretic peptides). The choice of different modalities depends on several factors: local availability and expertise, feasibility based on the patient's characteristics, and economic resources.

Immune checkpoint inhibitors (ICIs) targeting cytotoxic T-lymphocyte antigen-4 (CTLA-4) and programmed death-1/ligand-1 (PD-1/PD-L1) have transformed the treatment scenario of many different cancers, becoming a mainstay of treatment [6–8]. In fact, positive responses occur in a substantial fraction of patients and are frequently durable and even curative. Therefore, combined ICI blockade appears to

G. Manno · D. Di Lisi · G. Novo (✉)
Cardiology Unit, University Hospital Paolo Giaccone, Palermo, Italy

Department of Health Promotion, Mother and Child Care, Internal Medicine and Medical Specialties (ProMISE), University of Palermo, Palermo, Italy
e-mail: giuseppina.novo@unipa.it

A. Russo et al. (eds.), *Cardio-Oncology*, Current Clinical Pathology,
https://doi.org/10.1007/978-3-030-97744-3_6

51

further improve clinical outcomes compared with standard monotherapies [6–9]. Parallel to their efficacy as anticancer drugs, emerging evidences show immune-related adverse events involving the cardiovascular system in patients who are receiving ICI treatment [7, 10]. Although relatively rare, the cardiovascular toxicity of immunotherapy is serious and potentially fatal, and the true incidence in the general population of treated cancer patients is unknown. The main cardiotoxic complication is myocarditis, followed by coronary artery disease (atherosclerotic plaque rupture, acute myocardial infarction, vasculitis), conduction disease (atrioventricular block), noninflammatory LV dysfunction (heart failure and Takotsubo syndrome), and pericarditis. These adverse effects not only affect the quality of life of patients but also, above all, negatively affect the overall prognosis and occasionally force the interruption of life-saving drugs. In this context, the more precocious is the cardioprotective treatment, including drugs conventionally used to treat heart failure, the more effective is the damage reverse. For these reasons, there is a growing interest in the early assessment of cardiovascular damage induced by ICI treatment, through specific diagnostic programs [7]. ASCO 2018 recommends performing a 12-lead electrocardiogram (ECG) in the diagnostic workup of each patient receiving ICIs and suggests to consider troponin measurement especially in patients treated with combination immune therapies [11]. However, there is no consensus among the guidelines for the baseline cardiological evaluation and monitoring of asymptomatic patients. The ASCO and the ESMO guidelines recommend promptly performing a comprehensive cardiological evaluation when symptoms/signs of cardiovascular damage occur with ECG, troponin and additional tests such as brain natriuretic peptide (BNP), echocardiogram, and CXR. Further advanced exams such as stress test, cardiac catheterization, and cardiac MRI should be considered according to cardiologic consult [11, 12].

In this chapter, we will discuss the available diagnostic tools to detect cardiac immunotherapy damage and their integrated use. Figure 6.1 summarizes the main types of cardiac immunotherapy damage and the relative diagnostic tools available for their detection (adapted from Lyon et al. [6]).

Clinical and Electrocardiographic Evaluation

Clinical evaluation is always the cornerstone for overall baseline patient evaluation before starting ICI [3, 4, 6]. Physical examination (including blood pressure, heart rate, cardiological and pulmonary examination, peripheral pulses), exhaustive blood test panel (blood count, glucose, urea, creatinine, LDL and HDL cholesterol, triglycerides, fibrinogen, VES, sodium, potassium, calcium, magnesium, TSH, uric acid, homocysteine, HbA1c), should be performed in all patients [1–3]. Performing an ECG in the diagnostic workup of patients undergoing ICI is recommended. In fact, ECG might show prolonged PR interval, QRS axis deviation, bundle branch block, or second-degree or complete heart block [3, 4, 6]. Other changes in the ECG could be indicative of myocarditis (diffuse ST segment elevation) and pericarditis (PR depression and widespread saddle-shaped ST elevation). Moreover, although

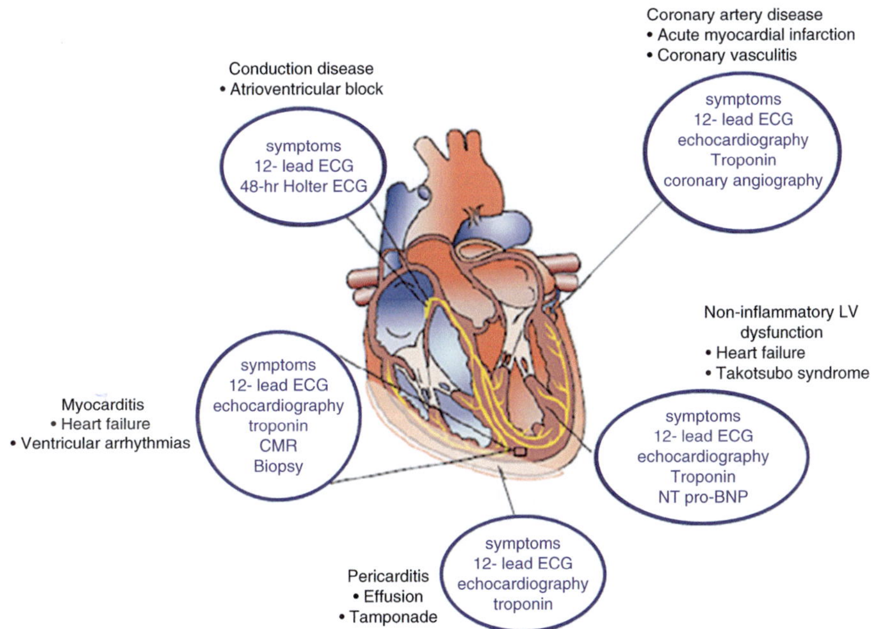

Fig. 6.1 Main type of cardiac immunotherapy damage and relative diagnostic tools available for the detection. (Adapted from Lyon et al. [7])

rarely, ICIs can be associated with myocardial infarction, characterized by chest pain, and new ischemic changes on ECG (e.g., ST elevation, ST depression, or T-wave inversion) [3, 13]. Moreover, 48-hour Holter ECG monitoring could be considered in patients who present symptoms such as palpitations, presyncope, or syncope [3, 14, 15]. In fact, ICI treatment can also be associated with atrioventricular conduction abnormalities, including heart block, bradycardia, and also atrial and ventricular tachyarrhythmias [14]. In severe cases, complete heart block and sudden cardiac death might occur [12, 15].

Echocardiography

Transthoracic echocardiography (TTE) is the most frequently used technique in clinical practice for monitoring anticancer therapy-related cardiac dysfunction (CTRCD) in cardio-oncology [3, 16–20]. In particular, two-dimensional (2D) TTE is the most commonly used technique for its repeatability, safety, wide availability, and low cost [3, 21]. Left ventricular volumes and left ventricular ejection fraction (LVEF) are the most widely used parameters to detect cardiotoxicity (CTX) [3, 18, 22]. 2D echocardiographic volume calculations use the biplane method of disc summation (modified Simpson's rule) as recommended by the European Association of Cardiovascular Imaging (EACVI) and the American Society of Echocardiography (ASE) [23]. Normal LVEF using modified Simpson's rule is 63% ± 5%, and LVEF in the range of 53–73% is classified as normal [23]. CTRCD is defined as a decrease in the LVEF of >10% points to a value less than the lower limit of normal in repeated studies and confirmed in a measurement repeated after 2–3 weeks [3, 18, 22]. Newer echocardiography techniques, using contrast echocardiography or 3D technology, have resulted in significant improvement in the accuracy of CTRCD detection [24–26]. Given the importance of assessment of regional wall motion abnormalities, the use of myocardial contrast is advisable when at least two contiguous segments are not adequately visualized to better outline the blood-endomyocardial interface, thus allowing an improved analysis of the geometry and function of the LV [25]. In fact, contrast echocardiography was found to have a strict correlation with LVEF measurement performed by cardiac magnetic resonance (CMR), the gold standard diagnostic for detection of LV volume [27]. Although 2D echocardiography is an excellent method, the concept of three-dimensional (3D) imaging has been envisioned by numerous investigators as a natural evolution of this technology [26]. Indeed, in patients with good image quality, 3D echocardiographic measurements are accurate and reproducible and should therefore be used if available [3, 25, 28]. One of the advantages of 3D echocardiographic volume measurements is that they do not rely on geometric assumptions [25, 28]. Despite the advantages of the standard echocardiography method, unfortunately, impairment of LVEF is detectable only after a considerable cell loss has taken place [17, 18, 29–31], thus making it too late for effective prevention. For this reason, new markers of systolic dysfunction have been investigated to earlier detect damage and predict cardiotoxicity [17, 18]. Deformation analysis imaging seems to be a promising tool to detect myocardial dysfunction at an earlier stage [30, 31]. A comprehensive echocardiographic evaluation including measurement of diastolic function, cardiac valves, and pericardium is recommended for cancer patients undergoing cardiological evaluation before starting potentially cardiotoxic drugs [3, 25]. Diastolic function is frequently impaired in cancer patients [22, 32]. In the oncological setting, the use of e′ velocity of the mitral annulus and E/e′ ratio using tissue Doppler imaging (TDI) remains questionable in consequence of changes in loading conditions associated with chemotherapy (e.g., anemia, diarrhea, nausea, and vomiting). However, an early reduction in the e′ velocity of the mitral annulus using TDI is very useful and indicative of initial diastolic dysfunction, and it remains reduced during and for several years after cancer treatment [33, 34]. Valvular heart disease may manifest in oncological patients treated with ICIs for different reasons such as pre-existing valve disease (and worsened after treatment) and mitral regurgitation secondary to annular dilatation or apical tethering due to CRDT or tricuspid regurgitation as consequence of right ventricle dysfunction and pulmonary hypertension [6]. Since pericarditis is one of the main complications of treatment with ICIs, a careful evaluation of the pericardium must be carried out [35, 36]. Pericarditis can occur in isolation, with typical pericardial pain, or can occur alongside myocardial involvement with perimyocarditis, or can be complicated by a pericardial effusion and possible cardiac tamponade. Pericardial effusion should be quantified and graded according to standard methods [37], and it is important to evaluate the presence of echocardiographic and Doppler signs of cardiac tamponade in this setting of patients [37].

Myocardial Deformation Imaging

LVEF reflects the volumetric variation of the ventricle during the cardiac cycle, but it is not a pure index of myocardial contractility. Furthermore, the decrease in LVEF is detectable when damage is considerable, and the possibility of recovery is reduced. It is not suitable as an early indicator of cardiotoxicity. Conversely, myocardial deformation analysis reflects the length variation of the myocardial fibers, and thus it is a measure of intrinsic contractility [31]. In this scenario, the analysis of the motion of speckles in the two-dimensional ultrasonic image offers a non-Doppler angle-independent objective analysis of myocardial deformation, with the possibility to quantify longitudinal, circumferential, and radial function and torsion. Speckle-tracking echocardiography (STE) has recently been demonstrated to be an accurate, feasible, and reproducible measure of cardiac function [38]. Particularly global longitudinal strain (GLS), evaluated as an average of the systolic strain value in all myocardial segments, can be used in the routine clinical practice and was shown to be a powerful prognostic marker. It has been demonstrated that a reduction in GLS precedes the reduction of LVEF in patients treated with anticancer drugs [39, 40]. The GLS in these studies provided superior prognostic information compared to LVEF. Percentage change from baseline higher than 15% in terms of GLS measurement has been recommended to detect subclinical cardiotoxicity in the setting of LV surveillance during anticancer treatment [25]. Moreover, recent publications suggest to use the changes in GLS (e.g., ΔGLS>15%) as a guide for an early cardio-protective intervention [41]. In a study of Awadalla et al. [42] it was retrospectively compared echocardiographic GLS by STE at presentation with ICIs myocarditis (cases, $n = 101$) to that from patients receiving an ICIs who did not develop myocarditis (control subjects, $n = 92$). Where available, GLS was also measured pre-ICIs in both groups. GLS was decreased in ICIs myocarditis and, compared with control subjects, was lower among cases presenting with either a preserved or reduced LVEF. Lower GLS was strongly associated with major adverse cardiac events (MACE) in ICI myocarditis presenting with either a preserved or reduced LVEF. Therefore, GLS represents a strong and useful adjunctive assisting tool for the evaluation of patients with cardiotoxic effect of ICIs. Technological progress in 3D echo has recently developed software that allows one to obtain a simultaneous quantitative assessment of all the strain components [24]. The main advantage of 3D STE corresponds to the possibility of analyzing the whole left ventricle from a unique data volume and considerably reducing the time of analysis in comparison with the more time-consuming 2D STE [43].

Nuclear Imaging and Cardiac Magnetic Resonance

Radionuclide angiography (MUGA) was referred to as the gold standard to evaluate left ventricle systolic function in patients undergoing chemotherapy for many years [44]. MUGA makes use of 99mTC-erythrocyte labelling enabling the visualization of the cardiac blood pool by γ-camera with electrocardiogram-triggered acquisitions. MUGA scan has been used since the 1970s as one of the first-line imaging modalities for baseline and serial assessment of LVEF for CTX. A problem with the use of this technique is the exposure of the patient to ionizing radiation. Furthermore, it does not permit evaluation of right ventricular function and atria and study of valves and pericardium [3]. For these reasons, it is a method rarely used today for the management of CTX. The need for a reliable and accurate detection method for early CTX has encouraged the introduction of second-line advanced imaging modalities into the evaluation of chemotherapy-treated patients, such as CMR [45]. This technique is able to accurately assess cardiac structure, function, and perform advanced myocardial tissue characterization, including perfusion, features which may facilitate the diagnosis, and management of CTX in cancer survivors [45]. In patients receiving ICI therapy, if myocarditis is strongly suspected, CMR including inflammatory sequences and late gadolinium enhancement is advisable, even if LVEF function is normal on echocardiogram [6]. If CMR is not available or is contraindicated, cardiac ^{18}F-fluorodeoxyglucose (^{18}F-FDG) PET/CT with appropriate fasting is helpful to detect myocardial inflammation or biopsy [46]. In a study by Mahmood et al. [47], 35 patients with ICI-associated myocarditis were enrolled from a multicenter registry with 8 sites and were compared to a random sample of 105 ICI-treated patients without myocarditis. The median time to the onset of myocarditis from the first ICIs was 34 days (interquartile range 21–75 days) with 81% presenting within 3 months of starting therapy. The LVEF was normal in 51% of cases of myocarditis. Thirty-one patients had a CMR study. In 20 cases, the diagnosis was made with the combination of an elevated troponin and the presence of late gadolinium enhancement on a CMR study in a pattern typical for myocarditis [48] and without evidence of coronary ischemia on standard testing.

Role of Biomarkers

In recent years, conventional biomarkers and emerging molecules have been studied in the context of CTX due to anticancer drugs, with the aim of ensuring an early diagnosis and follow-up [49, 50]. Currently, the most studied biomarkers for the early detection of cardiac damage induced by anticancer drugs are cardiac troponins (cTns) and natriuretic peptides such as brain natriuretic peptide (BNP) and N-terminal BNP (NT-pro-BNP) [47]. Troponin I and T (cTnI and cTnT) represent a sensitive marker of CTX in patients receiving anticancer drugs [49, 51, 52]. The elevation of troponin, particularly cTnI, was found to be earlier than the decline in LVEF, allowing the identification of patients at higher risk of developing cardiotoxicity [52]. Furthermore, the levels of cTnI evaluated over time have a very important prognostic value: persistently low values are associated with favorable outcome and do not require close follow-up [50–52]. Conversely, high levels of cTnI, especially if persistent 1 month after the end of treatment with high-dose anthracyclines, constitute a very reliable parameter for the identification of patients at high risk of CTX. In patients under ICI therapy, the cTns value is a valid diagnostic tool in case of suspected myocarditis or coronary artery disease. Even in milder CTX cases, a new increment of BNP or cTns allows the diagnosis of subclinical damage and helps in subsequent surveillance [6, 53]. Great attention must be paid to the differential diagnosis between increase of biomarkers secondary to CTX induced by ICIs or to non-toxicity-related cardiac conditions. In fact, biomarkers can increase in patients with advanced and metastatic cancer, particularly if they have pre-existing cardiovascular disease [6].

Role of Endomyocardial Biopsy

Although it is an invasive method, not free from complications, if myocarditis is strongly suspected, in patients with hemodynamic compromise or severe heart failure, endomyocardial biopsy is indicated [46, 48, 54, 55]. Beyond its diagnostic role, endomyocardial biopsy also plays a prognostic role and can drive therapeutic choices. In fact, current scientific evidence suggests immunosuppressive therapy only once a viral etiology has been ruled out with endomyocardial biopsy or when myocarditis is associated with known (non-cardiac) autoimmune disorders [55]. This latter consideration holds true for ICI-related myocarditis, in which treatment is mostly based on the use of glucocorticoids [11, 56].

Diagnostic Approach

There is no consensus among guidelines for the management of patients undergoing ICI treatment. Two strategies have been proposed:

- A first strategy suggests, for each patient, performing ECG and troponin measurement before starting treatment and therefore a recheck 48 hour after each administration.
- A second strategy suggests surveillance of cardiovascular symptoms/signs and check of ECG and troponin only in case they occur. If new symptoms/signs or significant troponin (>99th percentile of the upper reference value or significantly increase compared to baseline) or ECG abnormalities occur, with the suspicion of myocarditis, cancer treatment should be hold and prompt cardio-oncological evaluation performed [57].

In asymptomatic patient in the event of not significant increase (<3 times the upper limit of normal) of troponin values, an ECG and a new troponin check should be performed within 24–48 hours. If the ECG is negative and there is no troponin increase, treatment with ICIs can be continued, with troponin monitoring before each infusion. In case of a significant increase in troponin value, a temporary suspension of drug administration should be considered, as well as further measurement of the troponin within 24 hours, ECG, and cardiological counseling. The presence of pathological ECG alterations, together with the clinical evolution of the patient (onset of symptoms) will lead to the choice whether to hospitalize the patient [58].

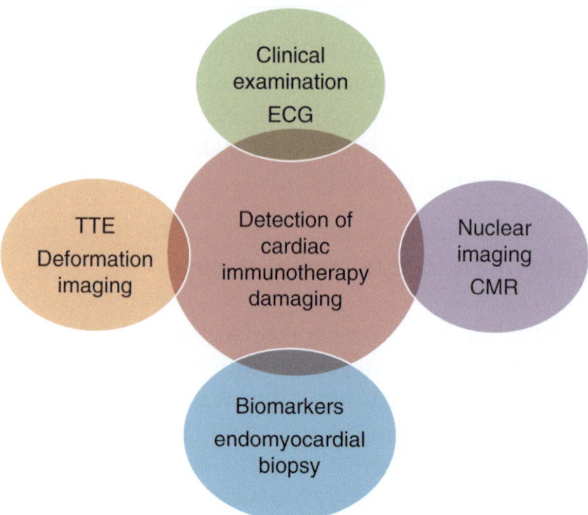

Fig. 6.2 Diagnostic tools for detection of cardiac damage induced by ICIs

In symptomatic patients, depending on the severity of the symptoms and according to cardiological counseling, hospitalization should be considered.

MRI should be considered in case of clinical suspicion of myocarditis. Coronary angiography/myocardial scintigraphy should be considered when acute coronary syndrome is suspected. Myocardial biopsy is an option in specific circumstances [58, 59].

Figure 6.2 shows the diagnostic tools available for detection of cardiac damage induced by ICIs.

Conclusion

CTX induced by ICI is a rare but serious complication with a relatively high mortality. Most CTX effects appear to be inflammatory in nature, and myocarditis represents the main complication. Although still relatively rare, the cardiovascular toxicity of immunotherapy is serious and potentially fatal, and the true incidence in the general population of treated cancer patients is unknown. Surveillance of the occurrence of signs/symptoms suggestive of cardiovascular adverse events is mandatory in patients treated with ICI. In the event that they occur, a prompt comprehensive cardiological evaluation is needed. An ECG and troponin surveillance at baseline and within 48 hours before each administration seem to be a reasonable approach.

References

1. Bray F, Ferlay J, Soerjomataram I, et al. Global cancer statistics 2018: GLOBOCAN estimates of incidence and mortality worldwide for 36 cancers in 185 countries. CA Cancer J Clin. 2018;68(6):394–424.
2. Biasillo G, Cipolla C, Cardinale D. Cardio-oncology: gaps in knowledge, goals, advances, and educational efforts. Curr Oncol Rep. 2017;19(8):55.

3. Zamorano JL, Lancellotti P, Rodriguez Muñoz D, et al. Authors/Task Force Members; ESC Committee for Practice Guidelines (CPG): 2016 ESC Position Paper on cancer treatments and cardiovascular toxicity developed under the auspices of the ESC Committee for Practice Guidelines: The Task Force for cancer treatments and cardiovascular toxicity of the European Society of Cardiology (ESC). Eur Heart J. 2016;37:2768–801.

4. Ewer MS, Ewer SM. Cardiotoxicity of anticancer treatments. Nat Rev Cardiol. 2015;12:620.

5. Tocchetti CG, Ameri P, de Boer RA, et al. Cardiac dysfunction in cancer patients: beyond direct cardiomyocyte damage of anticancer drugs: novel cardio-oncology insights from the joint 2019 meeting of the ESC Working Groups of Myocardial Function and Cellular Biology of the Heart. Cardiovasc Res. 2020;116(11):1820–34.

6. Wang DY, Salem JE, Cohen JV, et al. Fatal toxic effects associated with immune checkpoint inhibitors: a systematic review and meta-analysis [published correction appears in JAMA Oncol. 2018 Dec 1;4(12):1792]. JAMA Oncol. 2018;4(12):1721–8.

7. Lyon AR, Yousaf N, Battisti NML, et al. Immune checkpoint inhibitors and cardiovascular toxicity. Lancet Oncol. 2018;19(9):e447–58.

8. Wolchok JD, Chiarion-Sileni V, Gonzalez R, et al. Overall survival with combined nivolumab and ipilimumab in advanced melanoma. N Engl J Med. 2017;377(14):1345–56.

9. Motzer RJ, Tannir NM, McDermott DF, et al. CheckMate 214 Investigators. Nivolumab plus ipilimumab versus sunitinib in advanced renal-cell carcinoma. N Engl J Med. 2018;378(14):1277–90.

10. Moslehi JJ, Salem JE, Sosman JA, et al. Increased reporting of fatal immune checkpoint inhibitor-associated myocarditis. Lancet. 2018;391:933.

11. Brahmer JR, Lacchetti C, Schneider BJ, et al. Management of immune-related adverse events in patients treated with immune checkpoint inhibitor therapy: American Society of Clinical Oncology Clinical Practice Guideline. J Clin Oncol. 2018;36:1714–68.

12. Curigliano G, Lenihan D, Fradley M, et al. Management of cardiac disease in cancer patients throughout oncological treatment: ESMO consensus recommendations. Ann Oncol. 2020;31:171–90.

13. Nykl R, Fischer O, Vykoupil K, et al. A unique reason for coronary spasm causing temporary ST elevation myocardial infarction (inferior STEMI)—systemic inflammatory response syndrome after use of pembrolizumab. Arch Med Sci Atheroscler Dis. 2017;2:e100–2.

14. Gibson R, Delaune J, Szady A, Markham M. Suspected autoimmune myocarditis and cardiac conduction abnormalities with nivolumab therapy for non-small cell lung cancer. BMJ Case Rep. 2016;2016:bcr2016216228.

15. Behling J, Kaes J, Munzel T, et al. New-onset third-degree atrioventricular block because of autoimmune-induced myositis under treatment with anti-programmed cell death-1 (nivolumab) for metastatic melanoma. Melanoma Res. 2017;27:155–8.

16. Santoro C, Arpino G, Esposito R, et al. 2D and 3D strain for detection of subclinical anthracycline cardiotoxicity in breast cancer patients: a balance with feasibility. Eur Heart J Cardiovasc Imaging. 2017;18(8):930–6.

17. Di Lisi D, Madonna R, Zito C, et al. Anticancer therapy-induced vascular toxicity: VEGF inhibition and beyond. Int J Cardiol. 2017;227:11–7.

18. Di Lisi D, Leggio G, Vitale G, et al. Chemotherapy cardiotoxicity: cardioprotective drugs and early identification of cardiac dysfunction. J Cardiovasc Med (Hagerstown). 2016;17(4):270–5.

19. Novo G, Di Lisi D, Bronte E, et al. Cardiovascular toxicity in cancer patients treated with tyrosine kinase inhibitors: a real-world single-center experience. Oncology. 2020;98(7):445–51.

20. Zhao R, Shu F, Zhang C, et al. Early detection and prediction of anthracycline-induced right ventricular cardiotoxicity by 3-dimensional echocardiography. JACC: CardioOncol. 2020;2(1):13–22.

21. Picano E, Vañó E, Rehani MM, et al. The appropriate and justified use of medical radiation in cardiovascular imaging: a position document of the ESC Associations of Cardiovascular Imaging, Percutaneous Cardiovascular Interventions and Electrophysiology. Eur Heart J. 2014;35:665–72.

22. Zito C, Longobardo L, Cadeddu C, et al. Cardiovascular imaging in the diagnosis and monitoring of cardiotoxicity: role of echocardiography. J Cardiovasc Med (Hagerstown). 2016;17(Suppl 1):e35–44.

23. Lang RM, Badano LP, Mor-Avi V, et al. Recommendations for cardiac chamber quantification by echocardiography in adults: an update from the American Society of Echocardiography and the European Association of Cardiovascular Imaging. J Am Soc Echocardiogr. 2015;28(1):1–53.

24. Mor-Avi V, Lang RM, Badano LP, et al. Current and evolving echocardiographic techniques for the quantitative evaluation of cardiac mechanics: ASE/EAE consensus statement on methodology and indications endorsed by the Japanese Society of Echocardiography. Eur J Echocardiogr. 2011;12:167–205.

25. Plana JC, Galderisi M, Barac A, et al. Expert consensus for multimodality imaging evaluation of adult patients during and after cancer therapy: a report from the American Society of Echocardiography and the European Association of Cardiovascular Imaging. Eur Heart J Cardiovasc Imaging. 2014;15:1063–93.

26. Spallarossa P, Maurea N, Cadeddu C, et al. A recommended practical approach to the management of anthracycline-based chemotherapy cardiotoxicity: an opinion paper of the working group on drug cardiotoxicity and cardioprotection, Italian Society of Cardiology. J Cardiovasc Med (Hagerstown). 2016;17(Suppl 1):S84–92.

27. Jenkins C, Marwick TH. Baseline and follow-up assessment of regional left ventricular volume using 3- Dimensional echocardiography: comparison with cardiac magnetic resonance. Cardiovasc Ultrasound. 2009;7:55.

28. Lang RM, Mor-Avi V, Sugeng L, Nieman PS, Sahn DJ. Three-dimensional echocardiography: the benefits of the additional dimension. J Am Coll Cardiol. 2006;48(10):2053–69.

29. Dogdus M, Diker S, Yenercag M, Gurgun C. Evaluation of left atrial and ventricular myocardial functions by three-dimensional speckle tracking echocardiography in patients with euthyroid Hashimoto's thyroiditis [published online ahead of print, 2020 Sep 8]. Int J Cardiovasc Imaging. 2020; https://doi.org/10.1007/s10554-020-02011-3.

30. Banchs J, Jefferies JL, Plana JC, et al. Imaging for cardiotoxicity in cancer patients. Tex Heart Inst J. 2011;38:268–9.

31. Tarr A, Stoebe S. Early detection of cardiotoxicity by 2D and 3D deformation imaging in patients receiving chemotherapy. Echo Res Pract. 2015;2(3):81–8.

32. Di Lisi D, Bonura F, Macaione F, et al. Chemotherapy-induced cardiotoxicity: role of the tissue Doppler in the early diagnosis of left ventricular dysfunction. Anti-Cancer Drugs. 2011;22(5):468–72.

33. Sawaya H, Sebag IA, Plana JC, et al. Early detection and prediction of cardiotoxicity in chemotherapy-treated patients. Am J Cardiol. 2011;107:1375–80.

34. Nagy AC, Cserép Z, Tolnay E, et al. Early diagnosis of chemotherapy induced cardiomyopathy: a prospective tissue Doppler imaging study. Pathol Oncol Res. 2008;14:69–77.

35. Yun S, Vincelette ND, Mansour I, et al. Late onset ipilimumab-induced pericarditis and pericardial effusion: a rare but life threatening complication. Case Rep Oncol Med. 2015;2015:794842.

36. Heinzerling L, Ott PA, Hodi FS, et al. Cardiotoxicity associated with CTLA4 and PD1 blocking immunotherapy. J Immunother Cancer. 2016;4:50.

37. Adler Y, Charron P, Imazio M, et al. 2015 ESC Guidelines for the diagnosis and management of pericardial diseases: The Task Force for the Diagnosis and Management of Pericardial Diseases of the European Society of Cardiology (ESC)Endorsed by: The European Association for Cardio-Thoracic Surgery (EACTS). Eur Heart J. 2015;36(42):2921–64.

38. Cameli M, Mondillo S, Galderisi M, Mandoli GE, Ballo P, Nistri S, et al. Speckle tracking echocardiography: a practical guide. G Ital Cardiol (Rome). 2017;18(4):253–69.

39. Thavendiranathan P, Abdel-Qadir H, Fischer HD, et al. Breast cancer therapy-related cardiac dysfunction in adult women treated in routine clinical practice: a population-based cohort study. J Clin Oncol. 2016;34(19):2239–46.

40. Thavendiranathan P, Poulin F, Lim KD, et al. Use of myocardial strain imaging by echocardiography for the early detection of cardiotoxicity in patients during and after cancer chemotherapy: a systematic review. J Am Coll Cardiol. 2014;63:2751–68.

41. Santoro C, Esposito R, Lembo M, et al. Strain-oriented strategy for guiding cardioprotection initiation of breast cancer patients experiencing cardiac dysfunction. Eur Heart J Cardiovasc Imaging. 2019;20:1345–52.
42. Awadalla M, Mahmood SS, Groarke JD, et al. Global longitudinal strain and cardiac events in patients with immune checkpoint inhibitor-related myocarditis. J Am Coll Cardiol. 2020;75(5):467–78.
43. Pérez de Isla L, Balcones DV, Fernández-Golfín C, et al. Three-dimensional-wall motion tracking: a new and faster tool for myocardial strain assessment: comparison with two-dimensional-wall motion tracking [published correction appears in J Am Soc Echocardiogr. 2009 Jun;22(6):745-e1]. J Am Soc Echocardiogr. 2009;22(4):325–30.
44. Gottdiener JS, Mathisen DJ, Borer JS, et al. Doxorubicin cardiotoxicity: assessment of late left ventricular dysfunction by radionuclide cineangiography. Ann Intern Med. 1981;94:430–5.
45. Burrage MK, Ferreira VM. The use of cardiovascular magnetic resonance as an early non-invasive biomarker for cardiotoxicity in cardio-oncology. Cardiovasc Diagn Ther. 2020;10(3):610–24.
46. Laubli H, Balmelli C, Bossard M, et al. Acute heart failure due to autoimmune myocarditis under pembrolizumab treatment for metastatic melanoma. J Immunother Cancer. 2015;3:11.
47. Mahmood SS, Fradley MG, Cohen JV, et al. Myocarditis in patients treated with immune checkpoint inhibitors. J Am Coll Cardiol. 2018;71(16):1755–64.
48. Neilan TG, Shah RV, Abbasi SA, et al. The incidence, pattern, and prognostic value of left ventricular myocardial scar by late gadolinium enhancement in patients with atrial fibrillation. J Am Coll Cardiol. 2013;62:2205–14.
49. Novo G, Cadeddu C, Sucato V, et al. Role of biomarkers in monitoring antiblastic cardiotoxicity. J Cardiovasc Med (Hagerstown). 2016;17(Suppl 1 Special issue on Cardiotoxicity from Antiblastic Drugs and Cardioprotection):e27–e34. Review.
50. Meessen JMTA, Cardinale D, Ciceri F, et al. ICOS-ONE Study Investigators. Circulating biomarkers and cardiac function over 3 years after chemotherapy with anthracyclines: the ICOS-ONE trial. ESC. Heart Fail. 2020;
51. Cardinale D, Ciceri F, Latini R, et al. The ICOS-ONE trial. Anthracycline-induced cardiotoxicity: a multicenter randomised trial comparing two strategies for guiding prevention with enalapril: The International CardioOncology Society-one trial. Eur J Cancer. 2018;94:126–37.
52. Cardinale D, Biasillo G, Salvatici M, et al. Using biomarkers to predict and to prevent cardiotoxicity of cancer therapy. Expert Rev Mol Diagn. 2017 Mar;17(3):245–56.
53. Spallarossa P, Sarocchi M, Tini G, et al. How to monitor cardiac complications of immune checkpoint inhibitor therapy. Front Pharmacol. 2020;11:972. Published 2020 Jun 26
54. Escudier M, Cautela J, Malissen N, et al. Clinical features, management, and outcomes of immune checkpoint inhibitor-related cardiotoxicity. Circulation. 2017;136:2085–7.
55. Caforio AL, Pankuweit S, Arbustini E, et al. Current state of knowledge on aetiology, diagnosis, management, and therapy of myocarditis: a position statement of the European Society of Cardiology Working Group on Myocardial and Pericardial Diseases. Eur Heart J. 2013;34:2636–48.
56. Varricchi G, Marone G, Mercurio V, et al. Immune checkpoint inhibitors and cardiac toxicity: an emerging issue. Curr Med Chem. 2018;25(11):1327–39.
57. Alexandre J, Cautela J, Ederhy S, et al. Cardiovascular toxicity related to cancer treatment: a pragmatic approach to the American and European Cardio-Oncology Guidelines. J Am Heart Assoc. 2020;9(18):e018403.
58. Cardioncologia 2019. Raccomandazioni pratiche. Progetto speciale a cura del Gruppo di lavoro cardio-oncologia 2019 AIOM-AICO-ARCA-ICOS-SIAARTI-SIBioC-SIE. https://www.aiom.it/cardio-oncologia-2019.
59. Novo G, Di Lisi D, Manganaro R, et al. Arterial stiffness: effects of anticancer drugs used for breast cancer women. Front Physiol. 2021;12:661464. Published 2021 May 13. https://doi.org/10.3389/fphys.2021.661464.

Ettore Capoluongo

Introduction

In the last decades, although cancer mortality has started to significantly decrease and the number of survivors to continuously increase [1], cancer survivors still remain at higher risk for common cardiovascular events such as arrhythmias, heart failure, myocardial infarction, stroke, and valvular disease [1]. This can be related to cardiovascular toxicity (CTX) due to the use of such anticancer medications, particularly in those patients with other comorbidities or at increased risk for cardiovascular diseases. The prediction of these events is challenging, because of the lack of specific early biomarkers able to predict the onset of these side effects. Cardiac troponins (cTn) and natriuretic peptides (BNP) can represent valid biomarkers, but they are mainly useful for diagnosing rather than predicting a cardiovascular event. Nevertheless, these blood biomarkers are routinely used in cardiovascular medicine for diagnosis and risk stratification. Therefore, the use of these biomarkers is yet to be implemented in the early diagnostic pathway of cardiovascular toxicity in patients under anticancer therapy. In particular, anthracycline chemotherapeutic drugs can determine cardiomyopathy and heart failure (HF). Although those with breast cancer, leukaemia, lymphoma, and sarcoma [2] can benefit from anthracycline administration, the preventive cardioprotective strategies did not show significant positive effects in preventing adverse cardiac side reactions. Noteworthy, early detection of anthracycline-related cardiotoxicity by means of both biomarkers and

E. Capoluongo (✉)
Dipartimento di Eccellenza in Medicina Molecolare e Biotecnologie Mediche, Università Federico II, Naples, Italy

DAI – Medicina di Laboratorio e Trasfusionale, Azienda Ospedaliera Universitaria Federico II, Naples, Italy

CEINGE – Biotecnologie Avanzate, Naples, Italy
e-mail: capoluongo@ceinge.unina.it

© The Author(s), under exclusive license to Springer Nature Switzerland AG 2022
A. Russo et al. (eds.), *Cardio-Oncology*, Current Clinical Pathology,
https://doi.org/10.1007/978-3-030-97744-3_7

imaging, followed by rapid starting of cardioprotective strategies, could be more effective in terms of patient's management.

Using of each biomarker of anthracycline cardiotoxicity in this setting needs to be supported by clear evidence of their usefulness in clinical setting [1, 2].

Cardiac troponin (cTn) and N-terminal-pro-brain natriuretic peptide (NT-proBNP) are molecular biomarkers suggested to allow earlier detection of drug-induced CTX compared to other parameters such as left ventricular ejection fraction (LVEF) measurement [3]. Troponin is a biomarker of defined cardiomyocyte injury, whereas BNP is a marker of increased myocardial strain. Natriuretic peptides (NPs) are excellent markers of long-term cardiovascular dysfunction in asymptomatic patients [3]. Therefore, the data reported in the following paragraph will exclusively cover the biomarkers identified as powerful candidates in this regard.

Cardiac Troponins

Troponins T and I are released into circulation when a damage to cardiomyocytes occurs: elevated troponin levels indicate cardiac damage and left ventricular (LV) dysfunction.

Cardiac troponin assays (cTnT and or cTnI) are routinely utilized in cardiovascular or emergency departments to diagnose myocardial injury.

The large part of researches on relationship between cardiac troponins and cardiotoxicity have focused on early onset heart damage: the results of these investigations showed that early troponin elevation preceded variations in LVEF [4, 5].

Among lots of studies published in this setting, there are conflicting results mainly dependent on the type of cTn assay used: most of the previous and old assays employed a low-sensitive troponin, as compared to the most recent where highly sensitive cTns were involved [1]. The latter have high specificity for cardiac injury; therefore, it is possible to detect small amounts of myocyte damage and to provide treatments to minimize cardiotoxicity prior to the development of irreversible left ventricular dysfunction. However, the literature data are not always conclusive, particularly due to the different numerosity and type of patients analysed and to the lack of overimposability of the follow-up period investigated: in fact, there are no randomized controlled trials to establish whether the use of Tn assay may improve outcomes in patients suffering from cancer and heart disease. Currently, there is not enough data to guide the use of troponin in the evaluation of cardiotoxicity related to chemotherapy [6]. Using troponins has also been applied to monitor patients under an anthracycline regimen to stratify risk and early detection of cardiotoxicity, respectively. In a recent study enrolling more than 700 patients, who received high-dose chemotherapy, Tn serum levels were evaluated at 12, 24, 36, and 72 h and 1 month after chemotherapy [7]. The 70% of patients with a TnI < 0.08 ng/ml were associated to a negative predictive value of 99% for CV death, HF, life-threatening arrhythmia, or asymptomatic left ventricular ejection fraction reduction (LVEF) of 25% or more. Furthermore, with the persistence of a positive value of TnI, 1 month after chemotherapy, 84% of the patients presented a cardiac event. Nevertheless, the use of this cut-off in clinical setting has not yet been implemented in routine management of these cancer patients. However, a persistent elevation of TnI is associated with a greater degree of LV dysfunction and a higher incidence of cardiac events compared with transient elevations in Tn levels:

therefore, TnI remains the best biomarker to use in this setting [8]. Nevertheless, troponin resulted in a lower value in the early monitoring of cardiac toxicity caused by trastuzumab and/or lapatinib in patients with HER2-positive breast cancer [8], without any significant correlation between troponin, left ventricular dysfunction, and the survival rate of childhood cancer survivors.

Contrastingly, troponin T is mostly considered less useful since some studies have shown that this biomarker is not associated with myocardial infarction or coronary heart disease, but it is mainly linked to the risk of death, which is not directly ascribed to cardiovascular events [9]. Likewise, troponin elevation may guide an early treatment with enalapril, with cardioprotective significant consequences and a better patients' prognosis [1, 2]. Finally, also in paediatric population under anthracycline regimen, TnI was shown to be predictive cardiotoxicity [10, 11].

The effective implementation of these strategies must also be considered as many survivors fail to adhere to current screening guidelines, particularly in the paediatric setting [12]. The administration of cardioprotective strategies, along with the implementation of validated biomarkers for cardiotoxic risk identification, is crucial to continue to ameliorate both the short-term and long-term health of cancer patients [13]. Finally, as reported by Bracun et al., cTns are powerful predictors of LV dysfunction, especially in high-risk patients. Cardiac troponins are easy to measure and are available in almost all automated laboratory services: therefore, the authors suggest introducing cTn assay as a part of the standard blood draws in cancer patients treated with anticancer cardiotoxic drugs [14]. In this view, I completely agree with the authors about the need to harmonize the cut-offs in order to better distinguish the acute coronary syndrome, for which both the kits and laboratory cut-offs are designed, from cardiotoxicity. The latter does not still have a specific cut-off able to discriminate between the not-at-risk from the at-risk patients. Moreover, it has been demonstrated that cTn cut-points are gender- and age-specific: in fact, women and younger patients usually exhibit lower levels. Therefore, a smaller but significant deviation in cTn levels could have easily been missed in the published studies [14].

Brain Natriuretic Peptides

Brain natriuretic peptides (BNPs) are molecules released by ventricular cardiomyocytes that are capable to improve myocardial performance due to vasorelaxation and natriuresis [15]. The BNP prohormone, namely, N-terminal (NT)-proBNP, shows a similar longer half-life in plasma [15]. The increased serum levels of NT-proBNP are a diagnostic biomarker of heart failure and an independent risk factor for cardiovascular diseases [16]. BNP and the NT-proBNP are broadly assessed as important diagnostic and prognostic markers in established heart failure: in fact, the decrease of LVEF is the most common cardiotoxic event from anticancer regimens [4]. The capability of these natriuretic peptides to identify subclinical cardiac damage is still under investigation, and results published in the current literature are controversial. In fact, recent clinical trials and observational research using NT-proBNP as a biomarker of cardiotoxicity showed inconsistent results in terms of the correlation between elevated NT-proBNP and cancer treatment-associated heart failure [17]. Nevertheless, some studies demonstrated that BNP serum levels increase during antiblastic therapy and correlate with impairment of both diastolic and systolic function [18]. However, other studies did not confirm these findings [19, 20].

We think that there are some findings to take into account before definitively excluding the use of these biomarkers from the assessment of cardiotoxic risk. Particularly, a consistent number of publications analysed the role of NPs in different cancer populations. One study measured NP in an unselected cohort of 600 consecutive patients with first diagnosis of cancer, showing that the pre-oncology treatment of an elevated baseline NT-proBNP was a significant predictor of mortality risk (hazard ratio 1.54). In addition, a Kaplan–Meier survival rate of 67% versus 49% (in patients with normal NT-proBNP, $p < 0.001$) at a median of 25 months' follow-up was found [21]. It has also been reported that in patients with high NT-proBNP at 1-year follow-up, there was a significant decrease in LVEF. Furthermore, a strong correlation between the level of NT-proBNP at 72 h and the level of reduction of EF at 12-month follow-up was found, along with other markers of systolic and diastolic dysfunctions. Therefore, measurement of NPs not only helps identify patients who will develop cardiotoxicity but may also help determine the degree of cardiac dysfunction [22]. Another study showed that about 10% of cancer patients, under treatment with anthracyclines, experienced a cardiac event (such as LV dysfunction, symptomatic HF, arrhythmia, sudden cardiac death, or ACS) showed a BNP > 100 ng/L prior to the event [23]. Although with some limitations, particularly due to the absence of LV dysfunction in all patients with cardiotoxic effect, this study emphasizes the predictive value of BNP. In agreement with the previous findings on the adult population, also on paediatric patients, the measurement of BNP serum levels showed similar behaviours. In fact, in children under doxorubicin regimen, BNP raise resulted predictive of development of cardiomyopathy (with an associated LV dysfunction) as compared to healthy patients as controls, respectively [24].

There are some factors reducing the power of the published studies in this context: (a) the small sample size of the cohorts examined, (b) the retrospective design of research, (c) the lack of reference ranges, and (d) the different laboratory methods, where only recently we have available more robust chemistries as compared to 10–15 years ago. Regarding the modality of patient enrolment, we underline that (1) cohorts are generally small and unmatched among different studies; (2) different cancer types, under different chemotherapy regimens, were often evaluated; (3) a limited period of follow-up was observed; and (4) endpoint setting was not homogeneous between studies, with different cut-off values for BNP and timepoints for the serial BNP measurements. Correction by age of BNP values was not performed in overall studies, although it is very well established that in elderly people, levels of BNP are physiologically higher than in the younger population. On the contrary, renal dysfunction can also increase levels of NPs [25], whereas obesity is associated with lower levels of NPs. Finally, inflammation secondary to cancer has also been shown in some studies to cause elevation of NPs [25].

New Emerging Biomarkers

There are some other markers under investigation: the major part of these is not adopted in clinical setting as not only early predictors but also long-term predictors of cardiotoxicity. Table 7.1 shows the markers that are under investigation with a specific diagnostic value.

Table 7.1 Emerging biomarkers not still used in clinical setting

Biomarker (Ref.)	Main source	Mechanism effects	Effect on organ/tissue	Clinical outcome	Drug associated with cardiotoxicity
Myeloperoxidase [26]	Leukocytes	Atherogenic and pro-oxidant	Cardiac tissue damage	Risk of coronary artery disease and acute HF	Doxorubicin Trastuzumab
Galectin-3 [25]	Macrophages	Extracellular matrix turnover and fibrosis	Remodelling and development of cardiac fibrosis/fibroblast proliferation and collagen deposition	Predictive of mortality rate and HF	No association
Growth differentiation factor-15 [GDF-15] [27]	Most somatic tissues and abundant in placenta	Secreted in response to oxidative stress, inflammation, and injury seemingly to maintain cell and tissue homeostasis	Increased in some stress conditions: inflammation, myocardial ischemia, and cancer Immunomodulatory potential effect		No association
C-reactive protein (CRP)	Hepatocytes	Induced by interleukin-6	General Inflammatory marker	LFEV arrhythmia and cardiac arrest	Under debate, due to the limited specificity
Toll-like receptors (TLR2 and TLR4)	Mainly macrophages and dendritic cells	Natural immune response	Reduction of inflammatory, oxidative stress and cardiac apoptosis	Predictive of cardiac insufficiency caused by anthracyclines	Experimental data not validated in clinical setting
Arginine-NO metabolites [28] arginine, citrulline, ornithine, asymmetric dimethylarginine (ADMA), symmetric dimethylarginine (SDMA), and N-monomethyl arginine (MMA)	Most cells, endothelial cells, cardiac tissue	Play a central role in both cellular oxidative/nitrosative stress and endothelial dysfunction	Modulation of inflammatory stress in the heart Myofibrillar disarray	Anthracycline-induced cardiotoxicity Increase in arginine-NO metabolites in the early stage can predict the cardiac dysfunction caused by doxorubicin in the early stage [1]	Experimental data not validated in clinical setting

Conclusion

The individual response to antineoplastic treatments varies significantly, and the related risk for cardiotoxicity events is not very high and unpredictable. Therefore, the identification of at-risk patients remains challenging being difficult to predict which patient will benefit from such drug regimen. Literature is full of papers regarding the use of cardiovascular circulating biomarkers, particularly through the NPs and cTn assays, as useful tools to guide cardiovascular treatments. Nevertheless, these studies are limited by the small sample size and the heterogeneous populations. In addition, some confounding factors (age, gender, type of cancer, comorbidities, etc.) were not considered during the study comparisons. Therefore, there is no consensus on the use of biomarkers and cardiovascular treatments in cancer patients, although an urgent need for evidence regarding the usefulness of cardiac biomarkers in predicting LV systolic dysfunction in patients under antineoplastic regimens is desired [5].

We underline that only a moderate-level evidence supports the use of cardiac troponin and natriuretic peptides for risk stratification and early identification of anthracycline cardiotoxicity. Among some limitations of published studies, we can consider the following issues: (a) some studies used older chemotherapy treatments and are therefore not applicable to current anthracycline treatment schemes: (b) different biomarker assays have been used (low- and high-sensitive assays), with different cut-offs and performances; and (c) there is no consensus regarding the optimal timing and thresholds for troponin and NPs in anthracycline-treated patients [5, 14].

Noteworthy, in a very recent metanalysis [29], the overall sensitivity and specificity for the diagnostic value of troponins were 69% and 87%, respectively, with a negative predictive value of troponins in the prediction of LV dysfunction of 93%. In addition, regarding the different types of assays used in different studies, the present metanalysis did not find significant difference in predicting LV dysfunction. In detail, the high-sensitivity troponin assays resulted as not superior to conventional troponin analysis for the prediction of LV dysfunction, but this observation was limited due to unequal numbers of patients within both groups. In general, the sensitivity was 69% for high-sensitivity troponins vs. 75% for conventional troponins, while the specificity was 87% for high-sensitivity troponins vs. 89% for conventional troponins in identifying decreased LVEF. In most studies, also point-of-care Tn assays were used, but consistent data of comparison are not reported [29].

Alternative tools, based on multiparametric evaluation of individual cardiotoxic risk, able to combine serum biomarkers, cardiac risk factors, type of cancer treatment, and imaging parameters could be most likely accurate in identifying individuals at highest risk for cancer therapy cardiotoxicity [5, 14].

Therefore, before the routine implementation of these biomarkers, above all, as early predictors of cardiotoxic events, it is urgently necessary to improve generalized diagnostic protocols and standardize the pipeline for cardiotoxicity risk assessment, in order to facilitate the harmonization of the terminology and diagnostic criteria related to this risk, particularly when referred to the early stage of cardiotoxic events [14, 30].

Finally, although scientific data have generated a deep knowledge of both pathophysiology and clinical implications, homogeneous recommendations and operational requirements for cardio-oncology care are still limited [31]. It is important as the cardio-oncology cannot be merely based on laboratory tests or imaging alone, but it requires a robust infrastructure where high-quality medical care should be guaranteed by interdisciplinary cooperation, also in collaboration with family doctors in tight relationship with treating oncologist [31]. This means that serum or plasma biomarkers cannot neither work nor outperform alone.

References

1. Gai W, An J, Wang Z, Han X, Geng J, Liang Y, Guo Y. Research progress of biomarkers in early detection of chemotherapy-induced cardiotoxicity. Heart Fail Rev. 2020; https://doi.org/10.1007/s10741-020-09948-6.
2. Simões R, Silva LM, Cruz ALVM, Fraga VG, de Paula SA, Gomes KB. Troponin as a cardiotoxicity marker in breast cancer patients receiving anthracycline-based chemotherapy: a narrative review [J]. Biomed Pharmacother. 2018;107:989–96.
3. Zardavas D, Suter TM, Van Veldhuisen DJ, Steinseifer J, Noe J, Lauer S, et al. Role of troponins I and T and N-terminal prohormone of brain natriuretic peptide in monitoring cardiac safety of patients with early-stage human epidermal growth factor receptor 2-positive breast cancer receiving trastuzumab: a herceptin adjuvant study cardiac marker substudy. J Clin Oncol. 2017;35:878–84.
4. Tan LL, Lyon AR. Role of biomarkers in prediction of cardiotoxicity during cancer treatment. Curr Treat Options Cardiovasc Med. 2018;20(7) https://doi.org/10.1007/s11936-018-0641-z18. Nicol M, Baudet M, Cohen-solal A (2019) Co-morbidities subclinical left ventricular dysfunction during chemotherapy co-morbidities. Card Fail Rev 942:31–36
5. Upshaw JN. The role of biomarkers to evaluate cardiotoxicity. Current Treatment Options in Oncology. 2020;21:79.
6. Cardinale D, Sandri MT, Colombo A, et al. Prognostic value of troponin I in cardiac risk stratification of cancer patients undergoing high-dose chemotherapy. Circulation. 2004;109(22):2749–54. Large study demonstrating troponin as an early biomarker of cardiotoxicity with high dose chemotherapy
7. Ponde N, Bradbury I, Lambertini M, et al. Cardiac biomarkers for early detection and prediction of trastuzumab and/or lapatinib-induced cardiotoxicity in patients with HER2-positive early-stage breast cancer: a NeoALTTO sub-study (BIG 1–06).[J]. Breast Cancer Res Treat. 2017:1–8.
8. Welsh P, Preiss D, Hayward C, et al. Cardiac troponin T and troponin I in the general population: comparing and contrasting their genetic determinants and associations with outcomes. Circulation. 2019;139(24):2754–64. https://doi.org/10.1161/CIRCULATIONAHA.118.038529.
9. Cardinale D, Colombo A, Sandri MT, Lamantia G, Colombo N, Civelli M, et al. Prevention of high-dose chemotherapy-induced cardiotoxicity in high-risk patients by angiotensin-converting enzyme inhibition. Circulation. 2006;114:2474–81.
10. Thankavel PP, Mir A, Ramaciotti C. Elevated troponin levels in previously healthy children: value of diagnostic modalities and the importance of a drug screen. Cardiol Young. 2014;24:283–9.
11. Harris TH, Gossett JG. Diagnosis and diagnostic modalities in pediatric patients with elevated troponin. Pediatr Cardiol. 2016;37:1469–74.

12. Cox CL, Hudson MM, Mertens A, Oeffinger K, Whitton J, Montgomery M, Robison LL. Medical screening participation in the childhood cancer survivor study. Arch Intern Med. 2009;169(5):454–62.

13. Bansal N, Blanco JG, Sharma UC, Pokharel S, Shisler S, Lipshultz SE. Cardiovascular diseases in survivors of childhood cancer Cancer. Metastasis Rev. 2020;39(1):55–68.

14. Bracun V, de Boer RA. Troponins and natriuretic peptides to detect cardiotoxicity: useful biomarkers or paradise lost? Eur J Heart Fail. 2020;22(2):362–5.

15. Weber M, Mitrovic V, Hamm C. B-type natriuretic peptide and N-terminal pro-B-type natriuretic peptide – diagnostic role in stable coronary artery disease. Exp Clin Cardiol. 2006;11:99–101.

16. Ponikowski P, Voors AA, Anker SD, Bueno H, Cleland JG, Coats AJ, et al. 2016 ESC Guidelines for the diagnosis and treatment of acute and chronic heart failure: The Task Force for the diagnosis and treatment of acute and chronic heart failure of the European Society of Cardiology (ESC). Developed with the special contribution of the Heart Failure Association (HFA) of the ESC. Eur J Heart Fail. 2016;18:891–975. https://doi.org/10.1002/ejhf.592.

17. Wang YD, Chen SX, Ren LQ. Serum B-type natriuretic peptide levels as a marker for anthracycline-induced cardiotoxicity. Oncol Lett. 2016;11:3483–92. https://doi.org/10.3892/ol.2016.4424.

18. Novo G, Nugara C, Fava A, Mantero A, Citro R. Early detection of myocardial damage: a multimodality approach. J Cardiovasc Echogr. 2020;30(Suppl 1):S4–S10.2020r 10.

19. Sawaya H, Sebag IA, Plana JC, Januzzi JL, Ky B, Tan TC, Cohen V, Banchs J, Carver JR, Wiegers SE, Martin RP, Picard MH, Gerszten RE, Halpern EF, Passeri J, Kuter I, Scherrer-Crosbie M. Assessment of echocardiography and biomarkers for the extended prediction of cardiotoxicity in patients treated with anthracyclines, taxanes, and trastuzumab. Circ Cardiovasc Imaging. 2012;5(5):596–603.

20. Lenihan DJ, Stevens PL, Massey M, Plana JC, Araujo DM, Fanale MA, et al. The utility of point-of-care biomarkers to detect cardiotoxicity during anthracycline chemotherapy: a feasibility study. J Card Fail. 2016;22(6):433–8.

21. Pavo N, Raderer M, Hülsmann M, et al. Cardiovascular biomarkers in patients with cancer and their association with all-cause mortality. Heart. 2015;101(23):1874–80. https://doi.org/10.1136/heartjnl-2015-307848.

22. Sandri MT, Salvatici M, Cardinale D, Zorzino L, Passerini R, Lentati P, Leon M, Civelli M, Martinelli G, Cipolla CM. N-terminal pro-B-type natriuretic peptide after high-dose chemotherapy: a marker predictive of cardiac dysfunction? Clin Chem. 2005;51(8):1405–10.

23. Lenihan DJ, Stevens PL, Massey M, Plana JC, Araujo DM, Fanale MA, Fayad LE, Fisch MJ, Yeh ET. The utility of point-of-care biomarkers to detect cardiotoxicity during anthracycline chemotherapy: a feasibility study. J Card Fail. 2016;22:433–8.

24. Hayakawa H, Komada Y, Hirayama M, Hori H, Ito M, Sakurai M. Plasma levels of natriuretic peptides in relation to doxorubicin-induced cardiotoxicity and cardiac function in children with cancer. Med Pediatr Oncol. 2001;37(1):4–9.

25. Kajaluxy A, Alexander RL. The role of biomarkers in cardio-oncology. J Cardiovasc Transl Res. 2020;13:431–50.

26. Ky B, Putt M, Sawaya H, French B, Januzzi JL Jr, Sebag IA, Plana JC, Cohen V, Banchs J, Carver JR, Wiegers SE, Martin RP, Picard MH, Gerszten RE, Halpern EF, Passeri J, Kuter I, Scherrer-Crosbie M. Early increases in multiple biomarkers predict subsequent cardiotoxicity in patients with breast cancer treated with doxorubicin, taxanes, and trastuzumab. J Am Coll Cardiol. 2014;63(8):809–16.

27. Wischhusen J, Melero I, Fridman WH. Growth/differentiation factor-15 (GDF-15): from biomarker to novel targetable immune checkpoint. Front Immunol. 2020; https://doi.org/10.3389/fimmu.2020.00951.

28. Finkelman BS, Putt M, Wang T, Wang L, Narayan H, Domchek S, DeMichele A, Fox K, Matro J, Shah P, Clark A, Bradbury A, Narayan V, Carver JR, Tang WHW, Ky B. Arginine-nitric oxide metabolites and cardiac dysfunction in patients with breast cancer. J Am Coll Cardiol. 2017;70(2):152–62. https://doi.org/10.1016/j.jacc.2017.05.019.

29. Michel L, Mincu RI, Mahabadi AA, Settelmeier S, Al-Rashid F, Rassaf T, Totzeck M. Troponins and brain natriuretic peptides for the prediction of cardiotoxicity in cancer patients: a meta-analysis. Eur J Heart Fail. 2020;22(2):350–61.
30. de Boer RA, Meijers WC, van der Meer P, van Veldhuisen DJ. Cancer and heart disease: associations and relations. Eur J Heart Fail. 2019;21:1515–25.
31. Michel L, Rassaf T. Cardio-oncology: need for novel structures. Eur J Med Res. 2019;24(1):1. https://doi.org/10.1186/s40001-018-0359-0.

Management of Patients with Cardiac Toxicity: The Point of View of the Cardiologist

Andreina Carbone, Alessandro Inno, Fabian Islas, and Nicola Maurea

Introduction

Cancer patients receiving antiblastic therapy have an increased risk of developing cardiovascular complications, and the risk is even greater if there is a history of heart disease. The following serious complications have been reported: myocarditis (with impaired ventricular function and heart failure), pericarditis, accelerated atherosclerosis, arrhythmias, noninflammatory ventricular dysfunction (Takotsubo cardiomyopathy), vasculitis, and venous thromboembolism [1].

Immune checkpoint inhibitor (ICI) cardiovascular toxicity appears to be immune-mediated tissue damage. Cytotoxic T-lymphocyte-associated protein 4 (CTLA-4), programmed death-1 (PD-1), CTLA-4, and the PD-1/PD-L1 axis play a crucial role in the interaction between the immune system and the heart to limit tissue damage in case of inflammatory processes affecting cardiovascular tissue [2]. Recently, ICI therapy has been associated with atherosclerosis progression and cardiovascular events including myocardial infarction and ischemic stroke [3].

The American Society of Clinical Oncology (ASCO) has proposed general and organ-system-specific guidelines for the management of adverse events associated

A. Carbone
National Cancer Institute, IRCCS Pascale, Naples, Italy

A. Inno
Medical Oncology, IRCCS Ospedale Sacro Cuore Don Calabria, Negrar di Valpolicella, Verona, Italy
e-mail: alessandro.inno@sacrocuore.it

F. Islas
Cardiovascular Institute, San Carlo Hospital, Madrid, Spain
e-mail: fabislas@ucm.es

N. Maurea (✉)
Istituto Nazionale Tumori IRCCS Fondazione G. Pascale, Napoli, Italy
e-mail: n.maurea@istitutotumori.na.it

© The Author(s), under exclusive license to Springer Nature Switzerland AG 2022
A. Russo et al. (eds.), *Cardio-Oncology*, Current Clinical Pathology,
https://doi.org/10.1007/978-3-030-97744-3_8

with ICI [4]. In general, treatment of moderate or severe cardiotoxicity consists in interruption of the ICI and immunosuppression. Patients should be monitored during treatment for evidence of adverse events [4]. For cardiovascular events and complications, it is necessary to refer to the guidelines of the international cardiology societies.

Atherosclerosis and Cardiovascular Events

Animal and cellular studies have demonstrated that immune checkpoints, targeted PD-1, PD-L1, and CTLA-4 are critical negative regulators of atherosclerosis [5–7]. However, there are conflicting data about the possible role of ICIs, by inhibiting these key pathways in atherosclerosis, in the increase in atherosclerotic plaque and atherosclerosis-related cardiovascular events [8, 9]. Recently, Drobni et al. [3] evaluated whether exposure to an ICI was associated with atherosclerotic cardiovascular events in 2842 patients and 2842 controls, matched by age, a history of cardiovascular events, and cancer type. They showed that in the matched cohort study, there was a threefold higher risk for cardiovascular events after starting an ICI, and in the imaging study, the rate of progression of total aortic plaque volume was >threefold higher with ICIs. This association between ICI use and increased atherosclerotic plaque progression was attenuated with concomitant use of statins or corticosteroids [3]. Based on a complete nationwide cohort of patients, D'Souza et al. [10] showed that among patients with lung cancer and malignant melanoma, ICI-treated patients had increased rates of cardiac events. The 1-year absolute risk of cardiac events was about 7–10% in patients with lung cancer and malignant melanoma treated with ICI. The risk estimates were higher in these real-world data compared with pharmacovigilance studies [10]. In a meta-analysis of 59 studies (sample size: 21,664), in comparison to traditional chemotherapies, there was an increase in coronary ischemia over 6 months of follow-up among patients on ICIs [11]. In a large retrospective meta-analysis including >20,000 immune checkpoint-treated patients, 9.8% of treatment-related deaths were from cardiovascular events, including heart failure, myocardial infarction, and the development of a cardiomyopathy [12]. Older age, diabetes mellitus, higher blood pressure, male sex, prior radiation treatment, and a history of a cardiovascular event increased the risk for a cardiovascular event [3]. However, other potential mechanisms may be involved in the progression of atherosclerosis ICIs mediated, such as vasculitis and focal myocarditis misdiagnosed as acute myocardial infarction. ICI therapy may be considered as a modifier of cardiovascular risk; therefore, before ICIs, a comprehensive cardiovascular risk evaluation and optimization of preventive medical therapy with close monitoring thereafter are recommended.

More recent studies have demonstrated that acute coronary syndrome (ACS) may also be an adverse event from ICIs. Multiple cases of ACS have been found in association with ICIs [13, 14]; some cases have a cause-and-effect relationship with ICI use [15]. This adverse event likely results from ICIs changing the composition of atherosclerotic plaques, for example, by increasing the presence of T lymphocytes relative to macrophages [16]. In case of ACS, admission to the cardiology ward/intensive care unit is necessary. For the diagnosis and the treatment, follow the international guidelines for ST-elevation myocardial infarction [17] or non-ST elevation myocardial [18] infarction as appropriate and consider vasculitis if atherosclerosis is absent at coronary angiography. In case of ACS, ICI should be stopped, and the rechallenge should be considered when the patient is clinically stable and > 30 days post myocardial infarction with risk factor controlled [19].

Myocarditis and Heart Failure

Clinical Presentation

Myocarditis is the most common cardiac immune-related adverse event (irAE) during ICIs. Although this complication appears to be infrequent (with very variable incidence rates, reported to be between 0.1% and 1.14%, up to 2.4% in patients treated with combinations of anti-CTLA-4 and anti-PD-1) [20, 21], the mortality rate is high, about 40% of cases [22]. Myocarditis occurs early during treatment with ICI, usually within the first 3–4 administrations. It can manifest with an asymptomatic troponin elevation, fatigue, dyspnea, orthopnea, myalgia, palpitation, chest pain, lower extremity edema, lightheadedness, syncope, change in mental status, acute heart failure, pulmonary edema, and, in severe cases, cardiogenic shock, multiorgan failure, and ventricular arrhythmias [20, 21, 23]. Myocarditis may be asymptomatic, fulminant, progressive, or life-threatening [20, 24]. Acute heart failure may occur secondary to decreased cardiac function and diminished ejection fraction [20, 24]. Conduction abnormalities can include complete heart block [20] and arrhythmias. A variety of dysrhythmias may occur starting from mild forms (supraventricular tachycardia) and in extreme cases sudden death (ventricular tachycardias). Patients may also present with fatigue, malaise, myalgia, and/or weakness alone or in combination with more specific cardiovascular symptoms. Symptoms can often be masked by other irAEs (e.g., pneumonitis and hypothyroidism) [4].

Diagnosis

As the range of presentations is broad, any relevant alerting symptoms should trigger immediate testing with subsequent referral to cardiology/cardio-oncology specialists if necessary [21]. A prompt diagnosis is necessary so that ICIs should be immediately discontinued and an appropriate therapy can be started [21]. For the diagnosis, several tests are recommended: electrocardiogram, echocardiogram, biomarkers, cardiac magnetic resonance (CMR), and in some cases endomyocardial biopsy (EMB).

- *Electrocardiogram* is a not expensive test and should be performed at the onset of symptoms. In ICI-associated myocarditis, electrocardiogram findings include atrial and ventricular arrhythmias, conduction anomalies, ST-T wave alterations, QT prolongation, and Q waves, but in some cases, it may be normal.
- *Cardiac biomarkers*, such as troponin and B-type natriuretic peptide (BNP) or N-terminal-pro-BNP (NT-pro BNP), are useful in the diagnosis and prognosis of

myocarditis. Mahmood et al. [21] showed that peak troponin levels were associated to adverse cardiac events. When myocarditis is suspected, serum cardiac biomarkers should be measured, but a baseline troponin measurement before ICI initiation would be of important value to monitor marker changes.

- *Echocardiographic evaluation* is the first-line noninvasive imaging test in the assessment of ICI-associated myocarditis. Left ventricular ejection fraction (LVEF) and myocardial strain should be measured to assess cardiac dysfunction in the acute setting of myocarditis and during follow-up. The risk of adverse events was higher with a lower global longitudinal strain (GLS), regardless of LVEF [25]. Also, wall motion anomalies, diastolic function, and pericardial and valvular alterations should be investigated. Pericardial effusions have been reported in 7–17% of patients with ICI-associated myocarditis [21, 23].
- CMR is the gold standard noninvasive test for the diagnosis of myocarditis of other etiologies [26]. In ICI cardiotoxicity, late gadolinium enhancement (LGE) is present in only 23–48% of patients [23, 27], whereas it is present in approximately 80% of cases of non-ICI myocarditis [28]. However, systematic data on the use of CMR in ICI myocarditis are lacking, and larger studies are needed.
- EMB is the gold standard test for the diagnosis of myocarditis and is also useful for the definition of etiology. EMB should be performed in specialist centers after accurate evaluation of the benefits and the risks of the procedure. However, EMB is rarely a first-line test [29]. Data on EMB in ICI-associated myocarditis are scarce: lymphocytic filtrations and fibrosis were detected in a small sample of patients [23, 27].

According to international guidelines, myocarditis can be classified into three categories (definitive, probable, and possible), based on the results of diagnostic tests [29] (see Fig. 8.1), ECG, cardiac biomarkers, and echocardiogram including

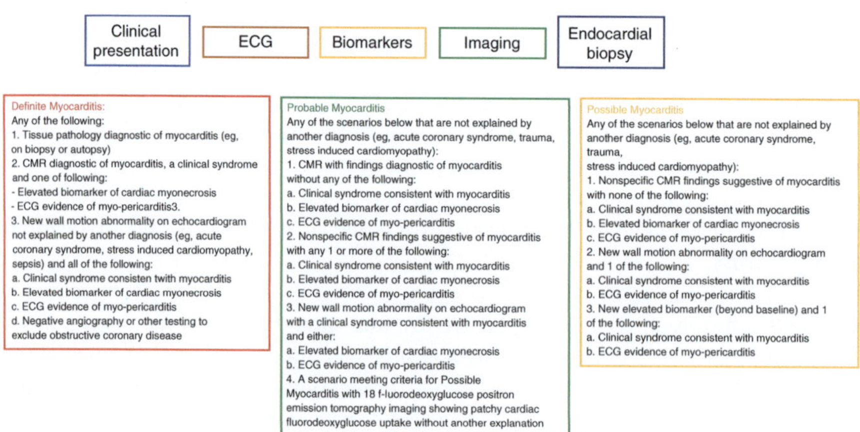

Fig. 8.1 Categories of myocarditis

Fig. 8.2 The figure represents an algorithm for the diagnosis of myocarditis. *ICI* immune checkpoint inhibitors, *CV* cardiovascular, *ECG* electrocardiogram, *BNP* brain natriuretic peptide, *GLS* global longitudinal strain, *CMR* cardiac magnetic resonance, *EMB* endomyocardial biopsy

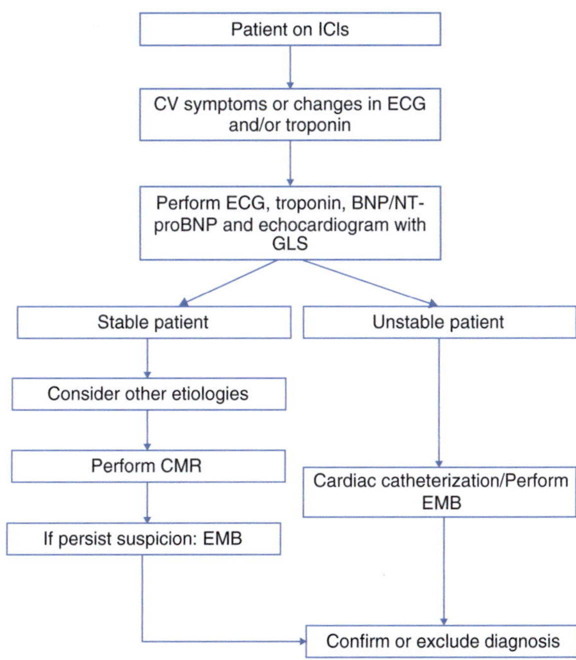

GLS as the initial tests to detect myocardial injury. For stable patients, CMR is the next line test, including standard tissue characterization and parametric mapping [30]. In cases of uncertainty, EMB should be considered, especially in patients in severe conditions and who are not responding to the therapies. For unstable patients (cardiogenic shock, cardiac arrest, or unstable arrhythmias), urgent cardiac catheterization should be considered to rule out ACS. Figure 8.2 is a proposed algorithm for the diagnosis of ICI-related myocarditis.

Management

There are no randomized trials testing treatment for ICI-associated myocarditis. The cornerstone of the treatment is immunosuppression [31]. When ICI-associated myocarditis is suspected, patients should be admitted to an oncology/medicine unit with telemetry or a cardiac care unit, depending on the severity of presentation. In unstable patients, discontinuing ICI and immunosuppression are recommended, without any delay [31]. Appropriate heart failure supportive therapy, with diuretics, renin-angiotensin-aldosterone system inhibitors, and beta blockers, should be promptly initiated. In cardiogenic shock, inotropes and cardiac mechanical support may be indicated [32]. Corticosteroids are the first strategy of immunosuppression in ICI-associated myocarditis [4, 19]. Intravenous corticosteroids (methylprednisolone 1000 mg/day in the acute phase, followed by oral prednisone (1–2 mg/kg)) are recommended, and a careful tapering should be started when the patient is stable,

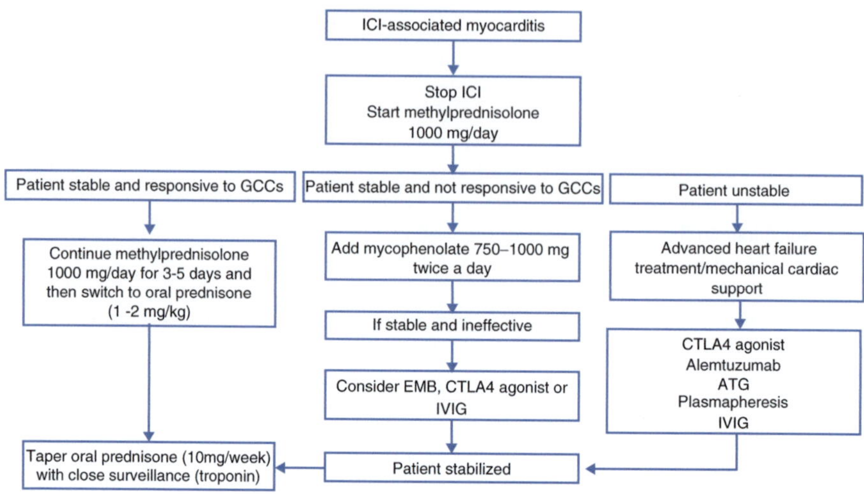

Fig. 8.3 Possible strategies of treatment in ICI-associated myocarditis

and the troponin begins to decline [4, 19]. Patients who do not respond to high-dose corticosteroids should be considered for other treatment options, such as abatacept (blocks CD86/ CD80-CD28 interaction), belatacept (a second-generation form of abatacept with increased binding affinity to CD86/CD80), alemtuzumab (CD52 monoclonal antibody), antithymocyte globulin (deplete T lymphocytes), or intravenous immunoglobulin (multiple activities) [31]. Infliximab should be used with caution in patients with heart failure [33]. It is recommended to definitively discontinue ICIs in cases of severe (grade 3) or life-threatening (grade 4) toxicities [19]. The risk of recurrence of myocarditis when patients are rechallenged with an ICI is unknown. ICI rechallenge should be avoided in patients with severe LV dysfunction, advanced conduction disease, or ventricular arrhythmias [19].

Figure 8.3 shows a possible algorithm for the management of ICI-related myocarditis.

ICI-Associated Pericarditis

Pericarditis (in isolated form or associated with myocardial involvement in a picture of perimyocarditis or myopericarditis) and/or pericardial effusion, up to a severe of cardiac tamponade, represents one of clinical manifestations of ICI-associated cardiovascular toxicity [19, 34]. The exact incidence of pericarditis during ICI treatment is unknown, varying from 0.1% to 7% in different series [34]. A retrospective observational analysis of the World Health Organization's pharmacovigilance database (Vigibase), published in 2018, reported 95 cases of adverse events of the pericardium in patients treated with ICI that appeared after a median of 30 days (interquartile range: 9–90 days) [18]. Pericardial toxicity was severe in most cases (81%), with a mortality rate of 21%. It was more frequent in patients treated with anti-PD1/anti-PDL1 than in those treated with anti-CTLA4. There were no significant differences in incidence between patients treated with monotherapy and those receiving ICI combinations. A systematic review of case reports and series, including a total of 28 cases of ICI-associated pericardial disease, showed that pericardial disease was reversible in the majority of cases (75%), although two deaths were reported. The majority of cases were life-threatening (G4, 53.6%) or severe (G3, 21.4%), requiring pericardiocentesis [34]. Pericarditis was treated with immunosuppression (high-dose steroids). ICIs were discontinued and then restarted in seven patients with no recurrence of pericarditis.

Table 8.1 shows the classification of pericarditis severity, according to the "National Cancer Institute. Common Terminology Criteria for Adverse Events" [35]. It's important to emphasize that pericarditis and pericardial effusion are not uncommon clinical manifestations in cancer patients. In fact, they have been reported to be between 0.1% and 4% [17]. These manifestations do not necessarily apply to immune-related toxicity, but may be related to other such causes as infections (more frequently viral, less frequently bacterial, including tuberculosis, and even more rarely, fungal or parasitic), cancer progression, autoimmune diseases, dysmetabolic alterations, post-traumatic damage, or toxicity from other antineoplastic drugs or radiotherapy [36].

Diagnosis

Shortness of breath is the most common symptom of ICI-related pericarditis [31]. Other symptoms consist of precordial pain, jugular venous congestion, and cardiogenic shock in cases of cardiac tamponade [31]. Diagnostic evaluation includes a detailed physical examination, ECG, and echocardiogram. ECG changes are

Table 8.1 Grade of pericardial disease according to NCI-CTCAE

	G1	G2	G3	G4
Pericarditis	Asymptomatic, ECG, or objective findings (e.g., pericardial rubs) consistent with pericarditis	Symptomatic pericarditis (chest pain)	Pericarditis with hemodynamic consequences (e.g., pericardial constriction)	Life-threatening consequences: urgent intervention indicated
Pericardial effusion	–	Asymptomatic, mild to moderate effusion	Effusion with hemodynamic consequences	Life-threatening consequences: urgent intervention indicated
Cardiac tamponade	–	–	–	Life-threatening consequences: urgent intervention indicated

present in up to 60% of cases and consist of new widespread ST elevation or PR depression. Echocardiography is the first-line test for the detection and study of pericardial effusion. CMR should reveal the concomitant presence of ICI-related myocarditis [31]. Chest X-ray, computed tomography (CT), positron emission tomography (PET), and CMR may help to differentiate ICI-associated pericarditis from malignant pericardial disease [36]. Analyses of pericardial fluid and pericardial/epicardial biopsies are usually performed in challenging cases and in cardiac tamponade [36].

Management

The following recommendations apply only to the treatment of immune-related pericardial toxicity; for pericarditis from other causes, refer to the main cardiological guidelines on this topic [36]. In case of grade 2 pericarditis with moderate (10–20 mm end-diastolic diameter with echocardiography) or severe (over 20 mm end-diastolic diameter with echocardiography) pericardial effusion, G3-G4 pericarditis, and cardiac tamponade, ICI should be discontinued. In cases of milder toxicity such as G1-G2 pericarditis or G2 with trivial (effusion visible only in systole) or mild (<10 mm in end-diastole) pericardial effusion [37], it is reasonable to continue ICI treatment in selected patients even in the absence of specific evidence and take into account their general conditions, disease status, and response to ICI. In the latter case, frequent clinical monitoring with periodic ECG is suggested (every 2–4 weeks or as agreed upon with the cardiologist in view of the clinical picture). ICI should be suspended in case of worsening or in case of an adverse event. Glucocorticoids can be administered. Prednisone (1 mg/kg/day) was used in most cases reported so far. The suggested treatment is prednisone or steroid equivalent of 1 mg/ kg/day, with subsequent slow scaling after the resolution of toxicity [38].

Aspirin/NSAIDs and colchicine are recommended in the guidelines of the European Society of Cardiology for the treatment of acute or relapsing pericarditis and for the treatment of pericardial effusion if associated with systemic inflammation; colchicine is not recommended in patients with renal insufficiency [36]. However, the role of these agents in the treatment of immune-related pericarditis and pericardial effusion has yet to be evaluated. Shaheen et al. [39] reported the case of a patient with non-small cell lung cancer who developed G3 pericardial effusion without cardiac tamponade while receiving nivolumab. The patient was managed with intravenous fluids to support the circulation, steroid therapy, and colchicine, which resulted in complete resolution of the effusion after 4 weeks; however, it returned when steroids were discontinued. Inno et al. [34] in a systematic review of case reports reported five patients treated with colchicine and/or NSAID with or without corticosteroids, achieving complete recovery in four cases and followed by effusion recurrence in one case.

The benefits of aspirin/NSAID or colchicine treatment in patients with immune-related pericardial toxicity remain uncertain. Nonetheless, based on the available evidence on the treatment of acute pericarditis and non-immune-related pericardial

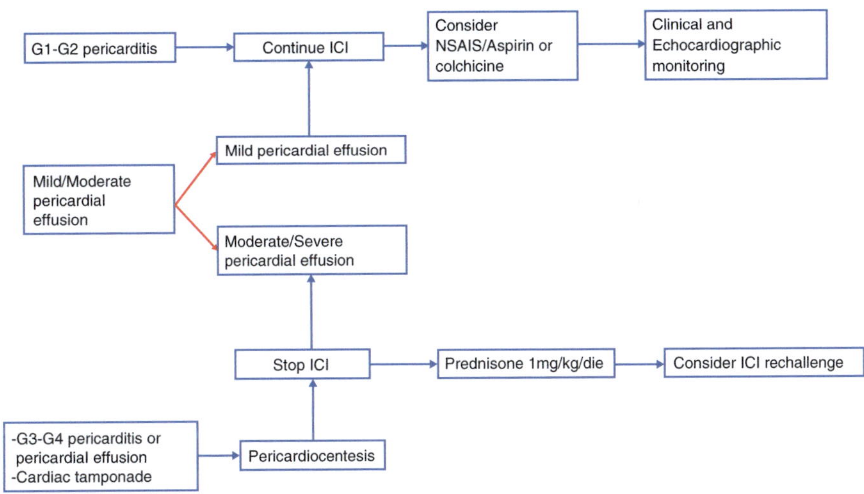

Fig. 8.4 Algorithm for the management of immunotherapy-related pericarditis/pleural effusion

effusion, and given the wide availability and favorable safety profile of these drugs, they may be considered for the treatment of patients with mild toxicity (pericarditis G1-G2 or trivial pericardial effusion). In case of hemodynamically significant pericardial effusion, a pericardiocentesis and/or other invasive procedures for the treatment of pericardial effusion may be used. Figure 8.4 is an algorithm for the management of immunotherapy pericardial complications.

Takotsubo Syndrome

Takotsubo syndrome (TS), also known as "stress cardiomyopathy" or "broken heart syndrome," is a transient form of left ventricular systolic dysfunction that mimics an acute coronary syndrome in patients not affected by obstructive coronary artery disease [40]. It affects postmenopausal women and adults and is usually attributed to emotional stress [40]. This syndrome has been associated with chemotherapeutic drugs, in particular 5-fluorouracil, combretastatin, pazopanib, and anagrelide [19, 41]. It has also been associated with immune checkpoint inhibitors [42]. A retrospective study showed that 14% of patients (4/29) with immunotherapy-related cardiotoxicity had TS [23, 43]. It has been suggested that TS could result from excessive production of catecholamine, microvascular dysfunction, or multivessel coronary artery spasm [44, 45]. It has been suggested that immune checkpoint inhibitors act directly on the coronary vasculature, thereby leading to multivessel coronary spasms. Another possible mechanism of action is the release of large amounts of epinephrine and norepinephrine from the adrenal gland and from postganglionic sympathetic nerves in the heart [19, 40]. The treatment of TS is mainly supportive: heart failure and arrhythmias are managed according to cardiology guidelines [18, 32]. Cardiac function will return to normal in most patients, although the in-hospital mortality rate is 2–8% [46]. In TS, it is important to pay attention to apical left ventricular thrombus related to apical ballooning and, if necessary, start anticoagulation treatment [40]. Lastly, both immunotherapy and TS may be associated with QT interval prolongation with the onset of life-threatening arrhythmias [40]. Further studies are needed to better understand the mechanisms underlying immunotherapy-related TS.

Arrhythmias

Patients with cancer may experience a wide spectrum of cardiac arrhythmias, namely, sinus tachycardia, bradyarrhythmias or tachyarrhythmias, and conduction defects, some of which may cause severe symptoms, become life-threatening, or require a change in the patient's treatment plan. Arrhythmias have been reported at baseline in 16–36% of cancer patients undergoing treatment and may be due to myocarditis and left ventricular ejection fraction, or it may be a primary disease manifestation [47]. Any type of supraventricular arrhythmia may arise acutely during or even after chemotherapy or radiotherapy, the most common being atrial fibrillation. The most common form of cancer-related atrial fibrillation is postoperative atrial fibrillation, particularly in patients undergoing lung resection [47]. ICI-associated myocarditis can present with various forms of arrhythmia including atrial fibrillation, ventricular arrhythmias, and conduction disease [23]. ICI-associated myocarditis may be associated with conduction defects consequent to inflammatory infiltrates encroaching upon the conduction system: electrocardiogram may show intraventricular conduction delay, interval prolongation, and eventually complete heart block [48].

Management

The treatment depends on the type of arrhythmias. Cardiology consult and electrophysiologist opinion are often indispensable [49, 50]. In general, the first approach is to consider discontinuing ICI treatment, depending on the severity of the condition, and then the use of conventional antiarrhythmic therapy (beta blockers, amiodarone, etc.) or cardiac pacing if necessary. In detail, in case of the following:

- New advanced conduction disease (second-degree or third-degree heart block): it is recommended to stop ICIs and consider intravenous methylprednisolone if any evidence of coexisting myocarditis (e.g., elevated troponin, cardiac MRI evidence). The cardiac treatment consists of emergency pacing.
- New atrial fibrillation: interrupt ICI therapy and consider rechallenge once stable and after myocarditis excluded. Immunosuppression is not recommended. Follow European Society of Cardiology guidelines for atrial fibrillation [51]. Consider direct current cardioversion and anticoagulation unless you get CHA2DS2-VASc score 0, contraindication, or short life expectancy.

- Ventricular tachycardia or ventricular fibrillation: emergency defibrillation (consider also beta blockers and amiodarone). Stop ICI and start intravenous methylprednisolone 500–1000 mg daily if myocarditis evident until clinically stable and troponin-negative followed by oral prednisolone 1 mg/kg once daily with weaning.
- Frequent ventricular ectopics (>1% of heart beats): interrupt ICI until myocarditis excluded and consider rechallenge after myocarditis is excluded. Consider β blocker, ECG, and Holter ECG surveillance if ICI treatment continues.
- New early conduction abnormality on ECG: continue ICI if Holter ECG excludes advanced heart block. Increase surveillance with ECG before each cycle of ICI.

Immunotherapy-Associated Vasculitis

ICI-associated vasculitis can affect vessels of various sizes but more frequently affects large vessels such as the temporal arteries [48, 52]. Temporal arteritis is an autoimmune and autoinflammatory disease of the aorta and its branches. Its manifestations are headache, jaw claudication, amaurosis fugax or diplopia, fatigue, fever, and weight loss with elevated inflammatory markers [48]. The diagnosis is performed with artery biopsy; Doppler ultrasonography is a noninvasive alternative [48]. The mechanism by which this phenomenon occurs may involve checkpoint pathway deficiency in the artery walls that predisposes to autoimmune attack [48]. It is recommended to interrupt the administration of checkpoint inhibitors and to start immunosuppressive treatment with intravenous methylprednisolone at 500–1000 mg daily for 3 days in patients with visual loss before switching to oral corticosteroids patients, whereas patients without visual loss should initiate immunosuppression with oral prednisone at 40–60 mg, given as a single daily dose [48].

Immunotherapy-Associated Thromboembolism

The onset rate of venous thromboembolism, which includes pulmonary thromboembolism and deep vein thrombosis, is four to seven times higher in cancer patients than in patients without cancer [52]. Arterial thromboembolism, which includes cerebral infarction, myocardial infarction, and peripheral embolism, is twice as high in cancer patients than in the general population [53]. The onset rate of arterial thromboembolism in cancer patients was reported to be 1.92% with the use of regimens containing cisplatin [54], 3.8% with ramucirumab [55], and 6.1% with bevacizumab [56]. It's possible that thromboembolism occurs consequent to the release of microvesicles rich in tissue factors from neoplastic cells that promote fibrin formation and platelet aggregation and formation of microthrombi [57]; however, the mechanism underlying venous thromboembolism during ICI administration in cancer patients remains unclear. Ando et al. [39] reported that the incidence of thromboembolism in patients receiving nivolumab and pembrolizumab was 7.1% and 10.8%, respectively. It's important to evaluate signs and symptoms of pulmonary embolism and/or deep venous thrombosis and to evaluate patients with suspected venous thromboembolism in patients undergoing immunotherapy [4]. Venous ultrasound for suspected deep venous thrombosis and computed tomography for suspected pulmonary embolism are recommended [4]. Also D-dimer can be considered for low-risk patients based on risk stratification as well as ECG, CXR, BNP, and troponin levels, as well as arterial blood gas testing according to the guidelines of societies of cardiology [1].

Screening and Surveillance

According to the American Society of Clinical Oncology (ASCO) [4] and the Italian Association of Oncology (AIOM) guidelines [58], the initial evaluation of patients with potential cardiovascular toxicity should include electrocardiogram and evaluation of basal troponin and brain natriuretic peptide (BNP) levels.

Electrocardiogram is recommended for all patients before and during treatment. It serves to detect signs of cardiac toxicity, including resting tachycardia, ST-T wave changes, conduction disturbances, QT interval prolongation, or arrhythmias. However, these ECG abnormalities are not specific and can be related to other factors [47]. The timing of cardiotoxicity surveillance using ECG and biomarkers should be patient-tailored in terms of their baseline cardiovascular risk and the cancer treatment protocol prescribed. Surveillance of troponin levels at regular intervals is recommended [59]. Data regarding the exact frequency of troponin monitoring and the appropriate patient population to screen are still lacking. The definition of specific patient populations at higher risk is under study and likely includes patients receiving combination ICI therapy [59]. Further data are also needed to evaluate the impact of cardiotoxicity surveillance on detecting myocarditis and subsequent treatment outcomes.

Conclusion

The development of novel therapies to treat cancer has led to increasing awareness of potential new cardiac toxicities, such as hypertension, arrhythmias, thrombotic complications, accelerated atherosclerosis, and immune-mediated myocarditis. Toxic myocarditis has emerged as a particularly dangerous complication associated with ICI use. ICI-induced myocarditis can be fulminant, with a high rate of mortality, but little is known about the clinical incidence, appropriate screening procedures, prevention, and treatment of this life-threatening toxicity. The mainstay of therapy for ICI cardiotoxicity has been corticosteroids, which have broad suppressive effects on the immune system and are associated with numerous side effects. More recently, other agents including antithymocyte globulin, mycophenolate mofetil, tacrolimus, and infliximab have been used in severe cases with some benefit. Larger studies are needed to understand the risk factors related to ICI cardiotoxicity and the optimal strategies to prevent this condition.

Table 8.2 summarizes the potential cardiac conditions associated with ICI administration and their management.

Table 8.2 Therapeutic strategies for ICI-associated cardiovascular toxicity

Cardiac toxicity	ICI strategies	Immunosuppression	Cardiac management
Myocarditis	Stop ICI	Intravenous methylprednisolone 500–1000 mg daily until clinically stable, followed by oral prednisolone 1 mg/kg once daily with weaning; second line: mycophenolate mofetil or infliximab; third line: antithymocite globulin or iv immunoglobulin	Diuretics, nitrates, ACE inhibitors, beta blockers
Advanced conduction disease (II-III-degree heart block)	Stop ICI	Consider iv methylprednisolone	Emergency pacing
Acute pericarditis without tamponade	Stop ICI and consider rechallenge when stable	Oral prednisolone 1 mg/kg once daily with weaning	Consider colchicine and NSAID
Cardiac tamponade	Stop ICI	Consider iv methylprednisolone 500–1000 mg daily until clinically stable, followed by oral prednisolone 1 mg/kg once daily	Emergency pericardiocentesis; consider colchicine and NSAID
Acute coronary syndrome	Stop ICI. Consider rechallenge when stable and > 30 days after myocardial infarction	Consider iv methylprednisolone if there is evidence of coronary vasculitis	Follow international guidelines of cardiology
Atrial fibrillation	Stop ICI. Rechallenge when stable	–	Follow international guidelines of cardiology
Ventricular arrhythmias	Stop ICI	Consider iv methylprednisolone	DC shock; antiarrhythmic drugs (amiodarone, beta blockers)
Takotsubo syndrome	Stop ICI. Consider rechallenge when stable	–	Follow international guidelines of cardiology
Vasculitis	Stop ICI	Consider iv methylprednisolone at 500–1000 mg daily for 3 days in patients with visual loss before switching to oral corticosteroids patients. Patients without visual loss should initiate immunosuppression with oral prednisone at 40–60 mg, given as a single daily dose	–

ICI immune checkpoint inhibitors, *ACE* angiotensin converting enzyme, *NSAID* nonsteroid anti-inflammatory drugs, *DC* direct current

References

1. Konstantinides SV, Meyer G, Becattini C, Bueno H, Geersing GJ, Harjola VP, et al. 2019 ESC guidelines for the diagnosis and management of acute pulmonary embolism developed in collaboration with the European Respiratory Society (ERS). Eur Heart J. 2020;41(4):543–603.
2. Baban B, Liu JY, Qin X, Weintraub NL, Mozaffari MS. Upregulation of programmed death-1 and its ligand in cardiac injury models: interaction with GADD153. PLoS One. 2015;10(4):e0124059.
3. Drobni ZD, Alvi RM, Taron J, Zafar A, Murphy SP, Rambarat PK, et al. Association between immune checkpoint inhibitors with cardiovascular events and atherosclerotic plaque. Circulation. 2020;142(24):2299–311.
4. Brahmer JR, Lacchetti C, Schneider BJ, Atkins MB, Brassil KJ, Caterino JM, et al. Management of immune-related adverse events in patients treated with immune checkpoint inhibitor therapy: American Society of Clinical Oncology Clinical Practice Guideline. J Clin Oncol. 2018;36(17):1714–68.
5. Fernandez DM, Rahman AH, Fernandez NF, Chudnovskiy A, Amir ED, Amadori L, et al. Single-cell immune landscape of human atherosclerotic plaques. Nat Med. 2019;25(10):1576–88.
6. Strauss L, Mahmoud MAA, Weaver JD, Tijaro-Ovalle NM, Christofides A, Wang Q, et al. Targeted deletion of PD-1 in myeloid cells induces antitumor immunity. Sci Immunol. 2020;5(43):eaay1863.
7. Gotsman I, Grabie N, Dacosta R, Sukhova G, Sharpe A, Lichtman AH. Proatherogenic immune responses are regulated by the PD-1/PD-L pathway in mice. J Clin Invest. 2007;117(10):2974–82.
8. Gelsomino F, Fiorentino M, Zompatori M, Poerio A, Melotti B, Sperandi F, et al. Programmed death-1 inhibition and atherosclerosis: can nivolumab vanish complicated atheromatous plaques? Ann Oncol. 2018;29(1):284–6.
9. Bar J, Markel G, Gottfried T, Percik R, Leibowitz-Amit R, Berger R, et al. Acute vascular events as a possibly related adverse event of immunotherapy: a single-institute retrospective study. Eur J Cancer. 2019;120:122–31.
10. D, Souza M, Nielsen D, Svane IM, Iversen K, Rasmussen PV, Madelaire C, et al. The risk of cardiac events in patients receiving immune checkpoint inhibitors: a nationwide Danish study. Eur Heart J. 2020.
11. Laleh Amiri-Kordestani JM, Cheng J, Tang S, Schroeder R, Sridhara R, Karg K, Connolly J, Beaver JA, Blumenthal GM, Pazdur R. Cardiovascular adverse events in immune checkpoint inhibitor clinical trials: A U.S. Food and Drug Administration pooled analysis. J Clin Oncol. 2018;36(15_suppl. 2020):3009–9.
12. Wang Y, Zhou S, Yang F, Qi X, Wang X, Guan X, et al. Treatment-related adverse events of PD-1 and PD-L1 inhibitors in clinical trials: a systematic review and meta-analysis. JAMA Oncol. 2019;5(7):1008–19.
13. Ferreira M, Pichon E, Carmier D, Bouquet E, Pageot C, Bejan-Angoulvant T, et al. Coronary toxicities of anti-PD-1 and anti-PD-L1 immunotherapies: a case report and review of the literature and international registries. Target Oncol. 2018;13(4):509–15.
14. Tomita Y, Sueta D, Kakiuchi Y, Saeki S, Saruwatari K, Sakata S, et al. Acute coronary syndrome as a possible immune-related adverse event in a lung cancer patient achieving a complete response to anti-PD-1 immune checkpoint antibody. Ann Oncol. 2017;28(11):2893–5.
15. Cautela J, Rouby F, Salem JE, Alexandre J, Scemama U, Dolladille C, et al. Acute coronary syndrome with immune checkpoint inhibitors: a proof-of-concept case and pharmacovigilance analysis of a life-threatening adverse event. Can J Cardiol. 2020;36(4):476–81.
16. Newman JL, Stone JR. Immune checkpoint inhibition alters the inflammatory cell composition of human coronary artery atherosclerosis. Cardiovasc Pathol. 2019;43:107148.
17. Collet JP, Thiele H, Barbato E, Barthelemy O, Bauersachs J, Bhatt DL, et al. 2020 ESC guidelines for the management of acute coronary syndromes in patients presenting without persistent ST-segment elevation. Eur Heart J. 2021;42(14):1289–367.

18. Ibanez B, James S, Agewall S, Antunes MJ, Bucciarelli-Ducci C, Bueno H, et al. 2017 ESC guidelines for the management of acute myocardial infarction in patients presenting with ST-segment elevation: The Task Force for the management of acute myocardial infarction in patients presenting with ST-segment elevation of the European Society of Cardiology (ESC). Eur Heart J. 2018;39(2):119–77.
19. Lyon AR, Yousaf N, Battisti NML, Moslehi J, Larkin J. Immune checkpoint inhibitors and cardiovascular toxicity. Lancet Oncol. 2018;19(9):e447–e58.
20. Johnson DB, Balko JM, Compton ML, Chalkias S, Gorham J, Xu Y, et al. Fulminant myocarditis with combination immune checkpoint blockade. N Engl J Med. 2016;375(18):1749–55.
21. Mahmood SS, Fradley MG, Cohen JV, Nohria A, Reynolds KL, Heinzerling LM, et al. Myocarditis in patients treated with immune checkpoint inhibitors. J Am Coll Cardiol. 2018;71(16):1755–64.
22. Wang DY, Salem JE, Cohen JV, Chandra S, Menzer C, Ye F, et al. Fatal toxic effects associated with immune checkpoint inhibitors: a systematic review and meta-analysis. JAMA Oncol. 2018;4(12):1721–8.
23. Escudier M, Cautela J, Malissen N, Ancedy Y, Orabona M, Pinto J, et al. Clinical features, management, and outcomes of immune checkpoint inhibitor-related cardiotoxicity. Circulation. 2017;136(21):2085–7.
24. Heinzerling L, Ott PA, Hodi FS, Husain AN, Tajmir-Riahi A, Tawbi H, et al. Cardiotoxicity associated with CTLA4 and PD1 blocking immunotherapy. J Immunother Cancer. 2016;4:50.
25. Awadalla M, Golden DLA, Mahmood SS, Alvi RM, Mercaldo ND, Hassan MZO, et al. Influenza vaccination and myocarditis among patients receiving immune checkpoint inhibitors. J Immunother Cancer. 2019;7(1):53.
26. Grani C, Eichhorn C, Biere L, Murthy VL, Agarwal V, Kaneko K, et al. Prognostic value of cardiac magnetic resonance tissue characterization in risk stratifying patients with suspected myocarditis. J Am Coll Cardiol. 2017;70(16):1964–76.
27. Zhang L, Awadalla M, Mahmood SS, Nohria A, Hassan MZO, Thuny F, et al. Cardiovascular magnetic resonance in immune checkpoint inhibitor-associated myocarditis. Eur Heart J. 2020;41(18):1733–43.
28. Aquaro GD, Perfetti M, Camastra G, Monti L, Dellegrottaglie S, Moro C, et al. Cardiac MR with late gadolinium enhancement in acute myocarditis with preserved systolic function: ITAMY study. J Am Coll Cardiol. 2017;70(16):1977–87.
29. Caforio AL, Pankuweit S, Arbustini E, Basso C, Gimeno-Blanes J, Felix SB, et al. Current state of knowledge on aetiology, diagnosis, management, and therapy of myocarditis: a position statement of the European Society of Cardiology Working Group on Myocardial and Pericardial Diseases. Eur Heart J. 2013;34(33):2636–48, 48a-48d
30. Ferreira VM, Schulz-Menger J, Holmvang G, Kramer CM, Carbone I, Sechtem U, et al. Cardiovascular magnetic resonance in nonischemic myocardial inflammation: expert recommendations. J Am Coll Cardiol. 2018;72(24):3158–76.
31. Zhang L, Reynolds KL, Lyon AR, Palaskas N, Neilan TG. The evolving immunotherapy landscape and the epidemiology, diagnosis, and management of cardiotoxicity: JACC: CardioOncology Primer. JACC CardioOncol. 2021;3(1):35–47.
32. Ponikowski P, Voors AA, Anker SD, Bueno H, Cleland JGF, Coats AJS, et al. 2016 ESC guidelines for the diagnosis and treatment of acute and chronic heart failure: The Task Force for the diagnosis and treatment of acute and chronic heart failure of the European Society of Cardiology (ESC) Developed with the special contribution of the Heart Failure Association (HFA) of the ESC. Eur Heart J. 2016;37(27):2129–200.
33. Mir H, Alhussein M, Alrashidi S, Alzayer H, Alshatti A, Valettas N, et al. Cardiac complications associated with checkpoint inhibition: a systematic review of the literature in an important emerging area. Can J Cardiol. 2018;34(8):1059–68.
34. Inno A, Maurea N, Metro G, Carbone A, Russo A, Gori S. Immune checkpoint inhibitors-associated pericardial disease: a systematic review of case reports. Cancer Immunol Immunother: CII. 2021;69:1327.

35. National Cancer Institute. Common terminology criteria for adverse events (CTCAE), version 5.0. Bethesda: National Cancer Institute; 2017. Available from: National Cancer Institute. Common Terminology Criteria for Adverse Events (CTCAE), Version 5.0. Bethesda: National Cancer Institute; 2017.

36. Adler Y, Charron P, Imazio M, Badano L, Baron-Esquivias G, Bogaert J, et al. 2015 ESC guidelines for the diagnosis and management of pericardial diseases: The Task Force for the Diagnosis and Management of Pericardial Diseases of the European Society of Cardiology (ESC)Endorsed by: The European Association for Cardio-Thoracic Surgery (EACTS). Eur Heart J. 2015;36(42):2921–64.

37. Klein AL, Abbara S, Agler DA, Appleton CP, Asher CR, Hoit B, et al. American Society of Echocardiography clinical recommendations for multimodality cardiovascular imaging of patients with pericardial disease: endorsed by the Society for Cardiovascular Magnetic Resonance and Society of Cardiovascular Computed Tomography. J Am Soc Echocardiogr. 2013;26(9):965–1012 e15.

38. Saade A, Mansuet-Lupo A, Arrondeau J, Thibault C, Mirabel M, Goldwasser F, et al. Pericardial effusion under nivolumab: case-reports and review of the literature. J Immunother Cancer. 2019;7(1):266.

39. Shaheen S, Mirshahidi H, Nagaraj G, Hsueh CT. Conservative management of nivolumab-induced pericardial effusion: a case report and review of literature. Exp Hematol Oncol. 2018;7:11.

40. Lyon AR, Bossone E, Schneider B, Sechtem U, Citro R, Underwood SR, et al. Current state of knowledge on Takotsubo syndrome: a position statement from the taskforce on Takotsubo Syndrome of the Heart Failure Association of the European Society of Cardiology. Eur J Heart Fail. 2016;18(1):8–27.

41. Chae YK, Chiec L, Adney SK, Waitzman J, Costa R, Carneiro B, et al. Posterior reversible encephalopathy syndrome and takotsubo cardiomyopathy associated with lenvatinib therapy for thyroid cancer: a case report and review. Oncotarget. 2018;9(46):28281–9.

42. Carbone A, Bottino R, Russo V, D, Andrea A, Liccardo B, Maurea N, et al. Takotsubo cardiomyopathy as epiphenomenon of cardiotoxicity in cancer patients: a meta summary of case reports. J Cardiovasc Pharmacol. 2021;78(1):e20–e29. https://doi.org/10.1097/FJC.0000000000001026. PMID: 34001727.

43. Ederhy S, Cautela J, Ancedy Y, Escudier M, Thuny F, Cohen A. Takotsubo-like syndrome in cancer patients treated with immune checkpoint inhibitors. J Am Coll Cardiol Img. 2018;11(8):1187–90.

44. Wittstein IS, Thiemann DR, Lima JA, Baughman KL, Schulman SP, Gerstenblith G, et al. Neurohumoral features of myocardial stunning due to sudden emotional stress. N Engl J Med. 2005;352(6):539–48.

45. Tsuchihashi K, Ueshima K, Uchida T, Oh-mura N, Kimura K, Owa M, et al. Transient left ventricular apical ballooning without coronary artery stenosis: a novel heart syndrome mimicking acute myocardial infarction. Angina Pectoris-Myocardial Infarction Investigations in Japan. J Am Coll Cardiol. 2001;38(1):11–8.

46. Gopalakrishnan M, Hassan A, Villines D, Nasr S, Chandrasekaran M, Klein LW. Predictors of short- and long-term outcomes of Takotsubo cardiomyopathy. Am J Cardiol. 2015;116(10):1586–90.

47. Zamorano JL, Lancellotti P, Rodriguez Munoz D, Aboyans V, Asteggiano R, Galderisi M, et al. 2016 ESC Position Paper on cancer treatments and cardiovascular toxicity developed under the auspices of the ESC Committee for Practice Guidelines: The Task Force for cancer treatments and cardiovascular toxicity of the European Society of Cardiology (ESC). Eur Heart J. 2016;37(36):2768–801.

48. Hu JR, Florido R, Lipson EJ, Naidoo J, Ardehali R, Tocchetti CG, et al. Cardiovascular toxicities associated with immune checkpoint inhibitors. Cardiovasc Res. 2019;115(5):854–68.

49. Brugada J, Katritsis DG, Arbelo E, Arribas F, Bax JJ, Blomstrom-Lundqvist C, et al. 2019 ESC guidelines for the management of patients with supraventricular tachycardia: The Task Force

for the management of patients with supraventricular tachycardia of the European Society of Cardiology (ESC). Eur Heart J. 2020;41(5):655–720.

50. Al-Khatib SM, Stevenson WG, Ackerman MJ, Bryant WJ, Callans DJ, Curtis AB, et al. 2017 AHA/ACC/HRS guideline for management of patients with ventricular arrhythmias and the prevention of sudden cardiac death: a report of the American College of Cardiology/American Heart Association Task Force on Clinical Practice Guidelines and the Heart Rhythm Society. Circulation. 2018;138(13):e272–391.

51. Hindricks G, Potpara T, Dagres N, Arbelo E, Bax JJ, Blomstrom-Lundqvist C, et al. 2020 ESC Guidelines for the diagnosis and management of atrial fibrillation developed in collaboration with the European Association for Cardio-Thoracic Surgery (EACTS): The Task Force for the diagnosis and management of atrial fibrillation of the European Society of Cardiology (ESC) Developed with the special contribution of the European Heart Rhythm Association (EHRA) of the ESC. Eur Heart J. 2021;42(5):373–498.

52. Goldstein BL, Gedmintas L, Todd DJ. Drug-associated polymyalgia rheumatica/giant cell arteritis occurring in two patients after treatment with ipilimumab, an antagonist of ctla-4. Arthritis Reumatol. 2014;66(3):768–9.

53. Navi BB, Reiner AS, Kamel H, Iadecola C, Okin PM, Elkind MSV, et al. Risk of arterial thromboembolism in patients with cancer. J Am Coll Cardiol. 2017;70(8):926–38.

54. Seng S, Liu Z, Chiu SK, Proverbs-Singh T, Sonpavde G, Choueiri TK, et al. Risk of venous thromboembolism in patients with cancer treated with Cisplatin: a systematic review and meta-analysis. J Clin Oncol. 2012;30(35):4416–26.

55. Fuchs CS, Tomasek J, Yong CJ, Dumitru F, Passalacqua R, Goswami C, et al. Ramucirumab monotherapy for previously treated advanced gastric or gastro-oesophageal junction adeno-carcinoma (REGARD): an international, randomised, multicentre, placebo-controlled, phase 3 trial. Lancet. 2014;383(9911):31–9.

56. Nalluri SR, Chu D, Keresztes R, Zhu X, Wu S. Risk of venous thromboembolism with the angiogenesis inhibitor bevacizumab in cancer patients: a meta-analysis. JAMA. 2008;300(19):2277–85.

57. Varki A. Trousseau's syndrome: multiple definitions and multiple mechanisms. Blood. 2007;110(6):1723–9.

58. https://www.aiom.it/linee-guida-aiom-gestione-della-tossicita-da-immunoterapia-2019/.

59. Waliany S, Lee D, Witteles RM, Neal JW, Nguyen P, Davis MM, et al. Immune checkpoint inhibitor cardiotoxicity: understanding basic mechanisms and clinical characteristics and finding a cure. Annu Rev Pharmacol Toxicol. 2021;61:113–34.

Management of Patients with Cardiac Toxicity: The Point of View of the Oncologist

Paola Zagami, Stefania Morganti, Paolo Tarantino, and Giuseppe Curigliano

Introduction

The field of immunotherapy has revolutionized the treatment of different types of cancer. At the beginning, the development of immunotherapy focused the primary attention on the immune activation axes; only the deeper understanding of the interactions between cancer, the tumor microenvironment, and the immune system has prompted the identification of the immunosuppressive mechanisms as the most important in the therapeutic field. The current clinical landscape of immunotherapy agents, in fact, uses both strategies to enhance the immune activation and dampen the immune suppression, thus facilitating the anticancer immune responses. The dynamics of interactions between cancer and immune system was originally referred to as the *theory of immune surveillance* (i.e., the immune system identifies cancerous and/or precancerous cells and kills them, thus preventing cancer occurrence). Over time, such a theory has been extended to the tumor "immunoediting" model with three phases: the elimination phase, in which the innate and adaptive immune system identify and destroy cancer cells (the actual "immune surveillance"); the equilibrium phase, in which the immune system maintains control over cancer cells with a balance between the production of immunostimulants (e.g., interleukin [IL]12) and immunosuppressants (e.g., IL23); and the escape phase, in which cancer cells manage to escape recognition and suppression by the immune system, leading to tumor progression [1]. Since such discoveries, the ability to evade immune suppression has become a tumor hallmark for cancer. Cancer cells evade

P. Zagami · S. Morganti · P. Tarantino · G. Curigliano (✉)
Division of Early Drug Development for Innovative Therapies, European Institute of Oncology IRCCS, Milan, Italy

Department of Oncology and Hemato-Oncology, University of Milan, Milan, Italy
e-mail: paola.zagami@ieo.it; stefania.morganti@ieo.it; paolo.tarantino@ieo.it; giuseppe.curigliano@ieo.it

immune responses by avoiding and dysregulating T-cell activation and recognition through a complex system of cellular and humoral mediators, collectively known as immuno-checkpoints [2]. One of the key mechanisms of immune escape is the enhanced expression of the membrane immuno-checkpoints programmed death ligand (PDL) 1 and PDL2 on cancer cells. The PDLs are capable to bind the programmed death protein (PD) 1 expressed on lymphocytes, antagonize T-cell reception (TCR), and CD28 co-stimulator signaling, thus inhibiting the activation of T cells. The immune checkpoint inhibitors (ICIs) like the anti-PD1, anti-PDL1, and anti-CTLA4 molecules are a novel class of anticancer agents designed to facilitate antitumor immune-response [3]. The US Food and Drug Administration (FDA) and the European Agency for Medicines (EMA) have approved a multitude of ICIs for several indications, both as single agents and in combination with chemotherapy, other immunotherapy agents, or TKIs.

The efficacy of ICIs to induce an anticancer response is not without side effects. The activation of the immune-response by ICIs can induce a systematic activation of the immune-competent cells, targeting normal tissue and organs, thus causing immune-related adverse events (irAEs). The most frequent irAEs such as rash, diarrhea, pneumonitis, and endocrine alterations are often self-limiting, reversible, and controlled by steroid therapy. Albeit less frequent, serious adverse events may occur, as observed with neurological and cardiovascular immune-mediated disorders. The ICI-related cardiotoxic effects are rare but serious, associated with significant morbidity, disability, and high mortality. Immune-related myocarditis is the most frequent and characterized among cardiovascular irAEs, but arrhythmias, heart failure, vasculitis, pericarditis, and also preclinical organ damage (e.g., elevated biomarkers of necrosis) represent alternative clinical manifestations that deserve proper attention. There are few prospective studies assessing the cardiotoxicity related to immunotherapy agents, largely missing key information about the characteristics, timing, and outcomes of irAEs [4]. The first two single case reports of fulminant myocarditis after administration of the ICI combination recalled the urgent need for further investigation into these specific toxicities, with a high potential to be fatal [5].

Cardiovascular irAEs occur in less than 1% of patients receiving immunotherapies. A retrospective analysis of the literature reported an incidence of ICI-associated myocarditis between 0.27% and 1.14%. These numbers are consistent with the data collected from the safety database of Bristol-Myers Squibb, including 20,594 patients (0.09%) treated with ipilimumab, nivolumab, or both, and with the WHO VigiBase pharmacovigilance database, which reported around 0.0038% myocarditis and around 0.0030% pericarditis of all irAEs [5, 6]. Mahmood and colleagues reported a prevalence of myocarditis related to ICIs of 1.14% (35 cases from 8 sites): 81% of these cases occurred within the first four cycles of immunotherapy (IT) [7]. The revision of the WHO database made by Moslehi reported similar timing of onset of immune-related (Ir)-myocarditis (within the first 6 weeks of IT) [9]. Similarly, Escudier et al. described the manifestation of 30 cases of cardiac irAEs within three ICI-therapy cycles [8].

In several studies, the combination of immunotherapy agents was related to higher mortality and risk for Ir-myocarditis compared to monotherapy therapies [5,

10, 11]. Given the rarity and the fatality of these irAEs, an early diagnosis and optimal management is needed.

Mechanisms of Action of Cardiovascular ICI Adverse Events

Mechanisms of cardiac toxicity have been characterized more extensively for chemotherapy and other antineoplastic agents [12, 13]. Conversely, the pathophysiology of cardiovascular irAEs is not completely understood but is likely to be immunological, differently from other anticancer drugs. The first evidence of a role of the immune checkpoint molecules in heart damages derives from studies conducted on PD1-knockout mice, which developed a spontaneous inflammatory cardiomyopathy with IgG deposition. Similarly, preclinical models of autoimmune myocarditis showed a myocardial injury with deposition of antibodies (IgG) against cardiac troponin I (cTnI) in PD1-knockout mice and myocardial infiltration of CD4 and CD8 T cells in CTLA4-depleted mice [14, 15]. Endomyocardial biopsies of patients with ICI-associated myocarditis also showed an infiltration of CD8 T cells, macrophages, and fibrosis with rare B cells, suggesting a direct myocardial injury mediated by the hyperactivation of cytotoxic T cells. Moreover, a mechanism of cross-reactivity through shared epitopes between tumor and myocardium can explain the T-cell infiltration of myocardium [5].

Similar immune-infiltrate of CD4 and CD8 T cells and macrophages were found in the pericardial sites and tumor of patients who developed IR pericarditis, mostly after thoracic irradiation [16]. The electrical conduction system of the heart can be affected during the ICI therapies, resulting in arrhythmias. Systemic inflammation states and local inflammation of the myocardium of the His-Purkinje conduction system can explain the mechanism of action for IR arrhythmias [17].

A noninflammatory pathogenesis has also been recognized for cardiac irAE in patients with pre-existing heart disease: in fact, the anti-PD1 molecules can accelerate myocardial dysfunctions through nonimmune mechanisms or worsen underlying Takotsubo syndrome [17]. Overall, T-cell responses against the myocardium are normally suppressed by a multitude of mechanisms of central and peripheral tolerance that can be inverted during immune-activating therapies for cancer. Moreover, the expression of PD(L)1 in cardiac normal tissues can suggest a role in homeostasis maintenance [17] (Fig. 9.1).

Myocarditis

Epidemiology

Myocarditis is the most frequently reported cardiac immune-related adverse event (irAE), with a prevalence between 0.09% and 1.14% [5, 7].

In 2016, Johnson et al. first reported two cases of fulminant myocarditis in patients receiving nivolumab plus ipilimumab [1]. Since then, several case reports

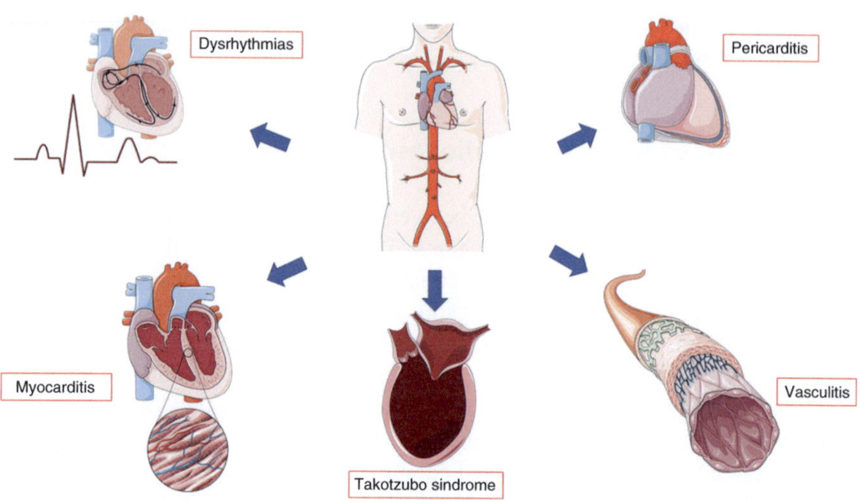

Fig. 9.1 Range of different cardiovascular toxicities associated with immune checkpoint inhibitors

and case series have been published, and the incidence of ICI-related myocarditis is expected to rise further as a consequence of the continuous expansion of ICI indications and growing awareness of this new clinical entity [8]. Even if rare, myocarditis is burdened by the highest mortality [6, 18].

Most cases occur early in the course of therapy, mainly within the first 1–2 months after the initiation of ICI [6–9]. Despite this, cases of late onset have also been reported [9], and an eventual diagnosis of myocarditis should be considered during all courses of treatment with ICIs.

The only well-established risk factor of ICI-related myocarditis is the administration of combination regimen (i.e., nivolumab and ipilimumab) [5, 11]. In patients receiving combination therapy, myocarditis was more frequently reported, was more severe, had a higher mortality, and was more often associated with non-cardiovascular irAEs like myositis and myasthenia gravis [11]. Although not proved, other theoretical risk factors include pre-existing cardiovascular and/or autoimmune comorbidities, concomitant or previous administration of cardiotoxic agents, genetic predisposition, concurrent non-cardiovascular irAEs (myositis and myasthenia gravis), and tumor-related factors (co-expression of antigens by cardiac tissue and tumor cells, activation of T-cell clones cross-reacting against cardiac self-antigens) [11, 17].

Physiopathology

Physiopathology of ICI-induced myocarditis is not completely understood. As shown by several pathology reports, ICI-associated myocarditis is mainly mediated by T cells and macrophages, with a minor to no role of B-cell immunity [5, 17].

T-cell infiltration is likely due to a cross-reactivity mechanism among antigens shared by the tumor and the heart, similar to what has been demonstrated in viral myocarditis [19]. Supporting this hypothesis, Johnson et al. performed T-cell receptor sequencing from tumor and cardiac infiltrates, observing the presence of high-frequency T-cell receptor sequences shared among cardiac and tumor infiltrating lymphocytes [5].

Interestingly, both CTLA4 and PD1/PDL1 axes demonstrated a crucial role in regulating cardiac immunity. PD1-deficient mice have been described to develop autoimmune dilated cardiomyopathy and premature mortality [20], and similarly, CTLA4-deficient mice were shown to develop severe multiorgan failure with autoimmune myocarditis with myocardial T-cell infiltration [21].

Moreover, cardiomyocyte PD-L1 expression was shown to be upregulated in several cases of cardiac stress and myocardial injury, including ischemia and left ventricular hypertrophy in preclinical models [22]. These findings suggest how the PD1/PDL1 axis can act as a brake to prevent inflammatory over-reactivity against cardiac tissue, while the administration of ICIs to susceptible patients can potentially unleash a strong autoimmune reaction by direct binding of ICI to cardiac tissues.

Clinical Presentation

The clinical syndrome associated with ICI-related myocarditis is variable and non-specific, spanning from asymptomatic and isolated elevation of cardiac biomarkers to severe decompensation with cardiogenic shock and end-organ failure. Most frequently reported symptoms include chest pain, palpitations, fatigue, and shortness of breath, mainly as manifestations of acute heart failure [5, 7, 9, 19]. However, up to 50% of patients may present with minor or no reduction in the ventricular ejection fraction [7]. Arrhythmias and pericarditis have also been described in patients with myocarditis [7, 11, 20], and other irAEs can co-occur, mainly myositis and myasthenia gravis [6, 9].

Laboratory and Imaging Findings

Elevation of serum troponin is recorded in almost all patients, even if this finding is not specific [7]. Cardiac troponin I should be preferred for assessing cardiac injury, given that troponin T may be elevated also in cases of myositis [11, 24]. Beyond the diagnostic value, troponin elevation also showed a prognostic role in the study published by Mahmood et al. [7].

B-natriuretic peptide (BNP) is also frequently increased in patients with ICI-related myocarditis but less specific than troponin [7, 11]. Overall, serum cardiac biomarkers should not be used to diagnose IR myocarditis, but be considered as supporting clinical elements in the context of a broader comprehensive cardiological assessment [11, 19].

Electrocardiogram (ECG) findings are nonspecific, but it should be performed to rule out alternative diagnosis such as acute coronary syndromes. Most frequently, the recorded alterations include PR interval prolongation, intraventricular conduction delay, and ST-T wave abnormalities [5, 19]. Several forms of arrhythmias have also been described, including atrial fibrillation, ventricular arrhythmias, premature ventricular contractions, and new heart blocks [9, 23].

Echocardiography should be performed to determine cardiac function and assess the status of the valvular apparatus and pericardium. Patients with severe ICI-related myocarditis usually present with a depressed left ventricular ejection fraction (LVEF), even if several cases of normal to minor reduction have been reported [7]. Alternative presentations include alterations of regional wall motion, abnormalities of diastolic parameters, and pericardial effusion [11, 19, 23]. It is still not clear if echocardiography should be performed or not as baseline investigation in patients candidate to receive ICIs, even if its role in monitoring eventual changes in cardiac function for patients with suspected cardiovascular toxicity is undoubtful [19].

Cardiac magnetic resonance (CMR) is the most specific imaging technique and allows to provide evidence of myocardial inflammation by showing concomitant myocardial edema and nonischemic injury [23].

The Lake Louise Criteria have been validated for the CMR diagnosis of myocarditis and were recently revised in 2018 (Table 9.1) [24]. These criteria rely on different sequences: T2 mapping or T2-weighted images to assess myocardial edema and T1 mapping, late gadolinium enhancement, and the extracellular volume fraction to assess nonischemic myocardial injury [24].

Cardiac ^{18}F-FDG PET/CT with appropriate fasting is a good alternative in cases of unavailability or contraindications to CMR [11, 23].

Endomyocardial biopsy (EMB) is the gold standard diagnostic test for myocarditis [11, 25]. Biopsy specimens should be analyzed by an experienced pathologist, and at least four to six samples should be obtained from different myocardial regions, in order to minimize false-negative results in cases of focal and patchy myocarditis [20, 24].

Table 9.1 Lake Louise Criteria for diagnosis of myocarditis by cardiac magnetic resonance

Main criteria (2 of 2): If both myocardial edema and nonischemic myocardial injury are identified, then CMR is highly suggestive of myocarditis with greater specificity. Having only 1 main criterion may still support the diagnosis of myocarditis in the correct clinical setting	(a) Myocardial edema Abnormal findings on T2 mapping or T2-weighted images
	(a) Nonischemic myocardial injury Abnormal findings on T1 mapping, LGE, or extracellular volume fraction
Supportive criteria Used alone, they are not diagnostic of myocarditis but may help support a diagnosis in the correct clinical setting that lacks 2 of 2 main criteria	(a) Pericarditis Evidence of pericardial effusion or abnormal LGE/T2 or T1 findings in pericardium
	(a) Left ventricular systolic dysfunction Regional or global wall motion abnormalities

Readapted from Ferreira et al. [24]

The Dallas criteria have been developed and validated as diagnostic pathologic criteria for myocarditis. They require two main components: inflammatory infiltrate and myocardial necrosis [19, 25]. Immune infiltrates mainly consist of CD8+ with CD4+ T cells and macrophages, while B cells are commonly absent [5].

A coronary angiography is frequently performed along with the endomyocardial biopsy in order to rule out an alternative diagnosis of coronary disease. Major complications to this procedure have been barely reported (<1%) [19].

Diagnosis and Management

All cases of patients presenting with signs and/or symptoms suggestive of immune-related cardiac toxicity should be promptly investigated and ICI withheld [26–28].

First-level assessment includes cardiac and inflammatory biomarkers, ECG, chest X-ray (CXR), transthoracic echocardiography, and cardiology consultation for consideration of second-level investigations, such as CMR and endomyocardial biopsy. The European Society for Medical Oncology (ESMO) guidelines suggest to perform EMB each time the diagnosis is highly suspected with otherwise negative workup [26]. If suspicion of myocarditis persists after first-level investigations, hospitalization is recommended [28]. Due to the possibility of life-threatening arrhythmias, patients should be monitored with continuous telemetry [27, 28].

Considering the relatively frequent co-occurrence of myocarditis and other forms of toxicities affecting the skeletal muscle, all patients with myositis and myasthenia gravis should have a cardiac assessment to investigate eventual myocardial involvement [27, 28].

Diagnosis of ICI-associated myocarditis is challenging, and several tests must be performed to rule out alternative diagnoses. On the other hand, it cannot be underestimated, given its high fatality rate. Bonaca et al. recently published a white paper aimed at establishing a uniform definition of myocarditis, to minimize underestimation and facilitate case ascertainment and reporting [23]. After a comprehensive diagnostic assessment, the probability of an ICI-associated myocarditis has been defined as definite myocarditis, probable myocarditis, or possible myocarditis, as reported in Fig. 9.2 [23]. As also reported in the fifth edition of the Common Terminology Criteria for Adverse Events (CTCAE v.5), isolated troponin elevation in asymptomatic patients is no longer sufficient for diagnosing myocarditis [29].

An additional classification categorizes ICI-associated myocarditis based upon its clinical severity as either fulminant, clinically significant, or subclinical. Fulminant myocarditis is referred to presentations with hemodynamic and/or electrical instability. Clinically significant non-fulminant myocarditis presents with signs, symptoms, and hemodynamic instability but does not meet criteria for fulminant. Finally, subclinical myocarditis refers to myocarditis not recognized or treated, with no evidence of clinical consequence [23].

Assessment of relatedness should be theoretically established using the nine Bradford Hill criteria [11, 30]. However, considering that many of these criteria are

DEFINITE MYOCARDITIS	PROBABLE MYOCARDITIS	POSSIBLE MYOCARDITIS
Pathology OR Diagnostic CMR + syndrome + (biomarker or ECG) OR Echo + syndrome + biomarker + ECG + negative angiography	Diagnostic CMR (no syndrome, ECG, biomarker) OR Suggestive CMR with either syndrome, ECG or biomarker OR Echo + syndrome (with either biomarker or ECG) OR Syndrome + PET and no alternative diagnosis	Suggestive CMR with no syndrome, ECG or biomarker OR Echo with syndrome or ECG only OR Elevated biomarker with syndrome or ECG and no alternative diagnosis

Pathology: Tissue pathology diagnostic of myocarditis(on biopsy or autopsy).

Cardiac Magnetic Resonance (CMR): diagnosis of myocarditis according to Lake Louise Criteria.

ECG: Arrhythmia, ST-T wave abnormalities, PR segment changes, or new arrhythmias (eg, new heart block or ectopy).

Biomarker: Elevated biomarker of cardiac myonecrosis(troponin I as the most specific).

Syndrome : Signs/symptoms associated with myocarditis such as palpitations, chest pain, acute or chronic heart failure, pericarditis, pericardial effusion.

Echocardiography (echo): New wall motion abnormality on echocardiogram not explained by another diagnosis.

Fig. 9.2 Definition of myocarditis. (Modified from Bonaca et al. [23])

Grade 1:	Grade 2:	Grade 3:	Grade 4:
Abnormal cardiac biomarker testing, including abnormal ECG	Abnormal screening testing with mild symptoms	Moderately abnormal testing or symptoms with mild activity	Moderately to severe decompensation, IV medication or intervention required, life-threatening conditions

Fig. 9.3 Grading of ICI-associated myocarditis according to ASCO guidelines [27]

often not feasible in patients, causal relationship should be defined considering temporality and after exclusion of alternative causes in the majority of cases [11].

Severity of myocarditis can be graded according to the American Society of Clinical Oncology (ASCO) guidelines (Fig. 9.3) [27]. Due to the potential for cardiac compromise, all grades warrant workup and intervention independently from severity, with the need for immediate and more intensive treatment increasing with grades.

According to American Society of Clinical Oncology (ASCO) guidelines, ICI therapy must be withheld in each patient with either suspicion or confirmation of ICI-associated myocarditis. Systemic prednisone or methylprednisolone is indicated at a high dose (1–2 mg/kg/day) for patients with mild to moderate (grade 2–3) myocarditis. For patients with more severe diseases (grade 3–4), higher doses of steroids (methylprednisolone at 1 g daily) are required, and eventually alternative immunosuppressors such as mycophenolate, infliximab, or antithymocyte globulin (ATG) should be administered in addition [27].

Considering management of ICI-associated myocarditis as suggested by National Comprehensive Cancer Network (NCCN) guidelines, intervention is indicated for severe (G3) and life-threatening (G4) myocarditis. The first is defined as "arrhythmia," significant echo findings without hypotension, cardiac markers > upper limit of normality (ULN)," and the latter as "arrhythmia, hemodynamic instability (hypotension/cardiomyopathy), cardiac markers >3xULN." In these cases, immunotherapy should be permanently discontinued and patients monitored in an intensive care setting. Methylprednisolone should be started at 1 g/day for 3–5 days, continued until recovering of cardiac function, and tapered over 4–6 weeks. In the absence of improvement within 24 hours on steroids, other immunosuppressive agents should be added, including ATG, infliximab, intravenous immunoglobulins, and mycophenolate. A transient pacemaker is advisable for patients with arrhythmia [28].

European Society Medical Oncology (ESMO) guidelines also recommend to permanently discontinue ICIs with any clinical myocarditis and promptly start high-dose corticosteroids (methylprednisolone 1000 mg/day followed by oral prednisone 1 mg/kg/day). Steroids should be than administered until resolution of symptoms and normalization of cardiac troponin, left ventricular systolic function, and arrythmias. In case of steroid refractory or myocarditis with hemodynamic instability, administration of other immunosuppressive therapies such as ATG, infliximab (except in patients with HF), mycophenolate mofetil, or abatacept is suggested. In addition to immunosuppression, patients with arrythmia, cardiomyopathy, and/or HF should receive appropriate therapy and cardiac support according to local guidelines [26].

Differently from most other irAEs, permanent discontinuation of ICIs is also recommended for mild (G1) toxicities, considering the elevated mortality and the absence of data about safety for the treatment rechallenge. In the absence of alternative therapies, readministration of ICI should be discussed case by case at a multidisciplinary level, and monotherapy with an anti-PD-1 agent with close monitoring should be preferred [26, 27].

It is still unclear whether a screening for myocarditis should be considered in patients candidate to receive a checkpoint inhibitor. No data are available supporting the use of baseline ECG or cardiac biomarkers to predict ICI-associated myocarditis or modify management, and the evaluation of surveillance strategies is limited by the rarity of these events. Some centers have implemented a minimal baseline assessment with ECG and troponins for patients at high risk (i.e., patients receiving a combination therapy), as per local guidelines [10, 27].

Pericarditis

Epidemiology

Pericarditis is a rare immune-related adverse events, mainly reported in literature as isolated case reports. In the largest observational study ever conducted to investigate the prevalence and characteristics of cardiotoxicities from ICIs, pericarditis was reported 95 times [6]. Most patients were affected by lung cancer and treated with anti-PD-1 or anti-PD-L1 as monotherapy (74/95). As previous reported for myocarditis, median time to onset was 30 days (9–90). Overall, 77 (81%) of 95 cases were reported as severe, with death occurring in 20 (21%) patients [6].

Concurrent irAEs were reported in 60 patients (63%), with pulmonary toxicities as the most frequently observed (40%). Only 4% of patients presented with concomitant myocardial involvement, and differently to what seen for myocarditis, musculoskeletal disorders was reported only in 5% of patients [6].

Predisposing factors are unknown. Only thoracic radiotherapy has been assumed as a potential risk factor, considering the relative higher frequency of patients with lung cancer [6, 16].

Pathophysiology

Pathophysiology underlying ICI-associated pericarditis is unclear. As reported above, previous cardiac irradiation seems to be a predisposing factor. Supporting this hypothesis, an increased mortality with combination of cardiac irradiation and anti-PD-1 antibodies has been observed in animal models, and preclinical studies have demonstrated a role of PD1 in modulating cardiac toxicity induced by radiotherapy [31].

Theoretically, administration of ICIs may also trigger the clinical manifestation of pericarditis of other etiologies, such as viral and connective ones, otherwise controlled by the PD-1/PD-L1 brake [16].

Histopathology findings of supposed ICI-related pericarditis showed a mild-to-strong immune infiltrate, consisting of CD4+ and CD8+ T cells, some CD68+ macrophages, and rare CD20+ B cells [16]. Quantitative immunofluorescence analysis revealed a similar immune marker expression profile (CD4, CD8, and CD20) between primary tumor and toxicity site, and no malignant cells were found in pericardial samples [16]. Macrophage infiltration assessed by CD68 protein expression was high in both pericardial sites and tumor sites at the time of toxicity development [16]. These evidences suggest a major role of macrophages in the pathogenesis of ICI-associated pericarditis, although the exact mechanism by which ICI can dysregulate macrophage function leading to the development of toxicity is still not clear.

Clinical Presentation

The main ICI-associated pericardial syndromes encompass pericarditis, pericardial effusion, and cardiac tamponade, ranging from mild and asymptomatic cases to severe life-threatening presentations [11].

Patients with pericarditis usually report chest pain relieved by forward position and present a typical friction rub on auscultation [32, 33]. Elevation of inflammatory markers (C-reactive protein, white blood cells, erythrocyte sedimentation rate) is common in patients with acute pericarditis, while cardiac biomarkers are above normal ranges in cases of concurrent myocardial involvement (peri-myocarditis) [32].

New PR depression and diffuse saddle-shaped ST elevation can be seen on ECG, while new pericardial effusion can be seen on echocardiogram. Cardiac MRI and ^{18}F-FDG PET/CT show evidence of active pericardial inflammation [11].

Diagnosis

Acute pericarditis is commonly diagnosed based on two of the following criteria: (a) chest pain relieved by sitting up and leaning forward, (b) pericardial friction/rub on auscultation, (c) characteristic ECG changes (new widespread ST elevation or PR depression), and (d) new or worsening pericardial effusion on echocardiogram [31]. These criteria apply to the more common idiopathic, viral, or autoimmune forms of pericarditis. It remains to be determined whether the prevalence of these manifestations differs between general pericarditis and ICI-associated pericarditis and if these criteria can apply also to the latter etiology.

Management

Initial diagnostic workup includes routine blood examination with cardiac biomarkers, chest X-ray, ECG, echocardiogram, and cardiac consultation. ICI should be promptly interrupted and high-dose corticosteroids started (1–2 mg/kg of prednisone) with subsequent taper [11].

Colchicine and NSAIDs can be administered according to guidelines of non-ICI-associated pericarditis. Emergency peri-cardiocentesis and hemodynamic support should be considered for the treatment of cardiac tamponade [16].

Acute Coronary Syndrome (ACS) and Myocardial Infarction (MI)

Epidemiology

Emerging data describes coronary complications as another potential form of ICI-related cardiovascular toxicity, including acute coronary syndrome (ACS) with myocardial infarction (MI).

Few data are available about immune-related ACS. Ferreira et al. described a case report of patient with lung cancer presenting coronary spasm during nivolumab treatment and identified other four cases of potential ICI-associated coronary toxicity reviewing pharmacovigilance registry and database available in literature [34].

ICI-associated myocardial infarction is a very rare irAE. According to a meta-analysis of 22 trials, only 2 events (incidence rate of 1%) occurred in patients with lung cancer receiving anti-PD1 or anti-PDL1 [35].

Physiopathology

The pathophysiology underlying ICI-associated ACS and MI is unknown. It has been hypothesized that, as already known for coronary syndrome, inflammation as a chronic condition or acute disease plays a crucial role in destabilizing atherosclerotic plaques. Thus, inflammation related to ICI therapy can induce or accelerate atherosclerosis and plaque rupture or, without atherosclerosis plaque, can develop a coronary spasm related to systemic inflammatory response syndrome [36, 37]. A form of vasculitis induced by ICI-mediated T-cell activation in coronary vessels has also been hypothesized as an alternative mechanism for ICI-mediated MI [17].

Clinical Presentation

Clinical manifestations of ICI-related ACS and MI are similar to those of other ACS. Patients often complain of chest pain, the most common symptom, which can radiate to the neck, left arm, shoulder, or upper abdomen. Elevated troponin is found on blood exams, and ECG shows ischemic changes as ST elevation/depression or T-wave inversion. Moreover, wall motion abnormalities in echocardiogram or cardiac MRI can be found. Thus, in patients receiving ICI who presented with elevated troponin with or without chest pain, an early differential diagnosis between myocarditis or MI is warranted.

Diagnosis

Diagnosis, treatment, and management of MI should follow ESC and AHA guidelines.

Diagnosis is based on clinical examination, ECG, and echocardiography. MI is commonly diagnosed in patients with elevated troponin associated with symptoms of ischemia and/or changes in ECG (ST segment changes, new left bundle branch block, or pathologic Q waves) and/or change in echocardiography. A definitive diagnosis of MI needs coronary angiography with the identification of a culprit occlusion or severe coronary stenosis [38, 39].

Management

After diagnosis of IR-MI, an immediate medical intervention is needed. If a coronary stenosis is identified, a percutaneous coronary intervention is indispensable, whether possible. The timing to proceed with percutaneous arterial procedure is related to pattern of presentation of MI, individual risk of acute cardiovascular event as assessed by standard scores, and the timing of onset of ischemia. A subsequent double antiplatelet therapy must be started as soon as possible [38, 39]. ICI have to be interrupted, and only after more than 30 days of clinical stability can rechallenge be considered, always in a multidisciplinary setting [17]. There is no evidence for the use of immunosuppressive therapy; indeed, some of them have been associated with an unfavorable cardiovascular profile [17].

Takotsubo Cardiomyopathy

Epidemiology

Takotsubo cardiomyopathy (TTS) is also known as stress-induced syndrome or transient apical ballooning syndrome. The incidence of Takotsubo syndrome is elevated in cancer patients treated with chemotherapy, which represents a major trigger for vasospasm [40]. In a retrospective study, 14% of cancer patients (4/29) experiencing cardiovascular irAE presented with a Takotsubo syndrome-like [9]. In the literature, six cases of TTS have been described in patients receiving pembrolizumab, ipilimumab, or combination therapy (tremelimumab and durvalumab or ipilimumab and nivolumab). Most of them were characterized by apical balloons, while only one was an "inverted" Takotsubo disease with akinesis in the basal and median segments of myocardium [41]. One case had an early onset (5 days) after starting ICI therapy, whereas the other five cases occurred after 8 weeks or more.

Pathophysiology

Differently from ICI-related IM or myocarditis, the pathophysiology of ICI-associated Takotsubo syndrome seems not to be related to inflammation or T-cell infiltration. Although the exact mechanism is still not defined, major hypothesis involves a direct action of ICIs on the coronaries, resulting in multivessel spasms, or a possible indirect injury on cardiomyocytes by catecholamine stress [42, 43].

Clinical Presentation

Clinical presentation ranges from asymptomatic to mild cases. It is characterized by a transient acute left ventricular dysfunction with apical akinesis and mid-left ventricular myocardium in the absence of coronary occlusion in angiography. ECG often shows transient abnormalities, and cardiac biomarkers' elevation (mainly BNP and pro-BNP and mild elevation of troponin) can also be detected [42].

Diagnosis

Diagnosis of TTS needs clinical examination, ECG, echocardiogram, cardiac biomarkers, and coronary angiography. Clinical manifestation can mimic acute coronary syndrome with reversible alteration on ECG (ST-segment elevation, ST depression, T-wave inversion, and/or QTc prolongation). The most characteristic sign is transient regional wall motion abnormalities, often in apical ventricular myocardium with specific form of balloon. Cardiac markers are elevated, mostly BNP and pro-BNP, with a smaller elevation for cardiac troponin. Diagnostic workup must include coronary angiography to rule out a coronary culprit lesion or stenosis [42].

Management

In patients with ICI-related Takotsubo disease, immune-therapy has to be promptly interrupted. In two reported cases, the use of high immunosuppressive therapy gave benefit, even if there are no recommendations available in this regard [43]. Cardioprotection with ACE inhibitors and beta-blockers can be considered to improve left ventricular function.

Dysrhythmias

Epidemiology

Dysrhythmias are rare irAEs that include various clinical manifestations. Almost one-third of patients experiencing immuno-related cardiotoxicity present with a form of dysrhythmia, with atrial fibrillation, ventricular arrhythmia, and conduction disorders, as the most frequently reported, occurring in 30%, 27%, and 17% of patients, respectively [9]. Such dysrhythmias can also be associated with left ventricular systolic dysfunction. Overall, the onset of dysrhythmias in patients experiencing immunotherapy-related cardiotoxicity is significantly associated with higher mortality [9].

Pathophysiology

The mechanism of immunotherapy-induced dysrhythmias is poorly understood. It is likely the consequence of immunotherapy-induced autoimmune myocarditis, with direct myocellular damage, tissue scarring, and disruption of the cardiac electrophysiology [44].

Diagnosis

Clinical examination and ECG are the cornerstones of diagnosis. A wide range of conduction abnormalities can be observed on the ECG, including tachycardia, conduction abnormalities, ST segment/T-wave abnormalities, QT prolongation, presence of Q waves, or atrial or ventricular arrhythmias [9]; nonetheless, none of these is specific to immunotherapy-related cardiotoxicity. Serum biomarkers (troponins, BNP) and trans-thoracic echocardiogram should also be requested when immunotherapy-related cardiotoxicity is suspected, with the latter being necessary to evaluate left ventricle function and the overall cardiovascular impact of the observed dysrhythmias.

Management

When immunotherapy-related dysrhythmias are diagnosed, depending on the severity of the event, patients should be admitted to an oncology unit/medicine unit with telemetry or cardiac care unit. Besides conventional guideline-based treatments for cardiac dysrhythmias, it is critical to discontinue immunotherapy treatment and initiate high-dose corticosteroids. In cases with a relevant cardiovascular impact and not responding to high-dose steroids, antithymocyte globulins or intravenous immunoglobulins can be considered, as well as infliximab or mofetil mycophenolate [45].

Vasculitis

Epidemiology

The term vasculitis identifies a heterogeneous group of diseases characterized by an inflammatory damage of the blood vessel walls. Although most commonly based on a primary immune disorder, immunotherapy-induced vasculitis has also been described in the literature, possibly due to the relevant role of checkpoint proteins in the pathophysiology of the disease. IR vasculitis can affect vessels of any size with different clinical manifestations, even if large vessels are most frequently involved and present as IR aortitis or IR temporal arteritis.

Vasculitis is an extremely rare irAE, almost never described in patients enrolled in clinical trials. A pharmacovigilance study reported vasculitis as 0.26% of all irAEs, with no significant difference between patients receiving anti-PD(L)1 or anti-CTLA4 antibodies [6].

Pathophysiology

Pathophysiology of immune-related vasculitis is still an object of study. Evidences about the role of checkpoint proteins in the pathophysiology of vasculitis are accumulating, with checkpoint molecule polymorphisms being associated with vascular T-cell activity in patients presenting with various forms of vasculitis [46]. Thus, checkpoint blockade may be responsible for a disruption of the physiological immune tolerance towards vascular components, inducing the release of cytokines, toxic mediators, and matrix metalloproteinases in arterial tissue by immune cells, ultimately resulting in vascular damage. To reinforce this hypothesis, temporal arteries with PD-1 and PD-L1 deficient expression promote T-cell infiltration in vessels and consequent arterial wall inflammation. The use of ICI mimes this immune environment [11].

Clinical Presentation

Clinical presentation depends on the size of the vessels affected. For example, temporal arteritis is characterized by headache, amaurosis, fatigue, and fever, while the involvement of small vessels such as the coronaries can present as acute coronary syndrome, MI, or Takotsubo syndrome [11].

Diagnosis

Diagnosis is based on traditional algorithms for primary vasculitis and includes clinical examination, blood tests with inflammatory markers, auto-antibodies (e.g., p- and c-ANCA), complement components, and imaging tests when indicated.

Inflammatory markers such as C-reactive protein and erythrocyte sedimentation rate are often elevated. Color doppler ultrasound is often performed, even if its utility for etiology investigation is doubtful. Pathology examination of cutaneous biopsies is often required as part of the diagnostic algorithm to demonstrate CD4 T-cell infiltration. It is particularly challenging to differentiate an immunotherapy-related vasculitis from a paraneoplastic vasculitis, which may present with overlapping manifestations [47].

Management

Due to the rarity of the event, specific treatment guidelines for immunotherapy-related vasculitis have yet to be defined. Given the potential severity of the manifestation, immunotherapy interruption and initiation of high-dose corticosteroids are generally recommended, in particular for temporal arteritis because of the risk of visual loss. A systematic review of all published cases of ICI-related vasculitis reported the resolution of symptoms in all patients, with either withholding of ICI and/or administration of glucocorticoids [48]. However, in case of steroid-refractory vasculitis, a variety of other immunosuppressive strategies can be evaluated, including azathioprine, mycophenolate mofetil (MMF), or intravenous cyclophosphamide, with different indications and schedules according to the specific type of vasculitis [49].

Cardiotoxicity Related to New Immunotherapy (CAR T Cell)

Epidemiology

Besides, an emerging immunotherapeutic strategy is represented by adoptive T-cell therapy (ACT), mostly implemented for the treatment of hematological malignancies but also for the treatment of solid tumors [50]. In this context, cardiotoxicity has been described as an effect of the cytokine release syndrome (CRS) induced by the treatment itself [51]. The incidence of cardiotoxicity induced by ACT-related cytokine storm is relatively high, with up to 27% of the patients experiencing G3–4 hypotension during treatment [52]. Other common symptoms observed in the course of ACT-related cardiotoxicity are tachycardia, arrhythmias, and, in the most severe cases, cardiopulmonary arrest.

Pathophysiology

A cardiomyopathy induced by systemic inflammatory response syndrome, related to cytokine storm, is the most common cause of left ventricle disfunction in the context of ACT treatment. Less frequently, off-target cross-reactivity of affinity-enhanced T cells can be responsible for cardiotoxicity through the immune targeting of cardiomyocytic peptides which resemble tumor antigens [53].

Diagnosis

The diagnosis of ACT/CRS-related cardiotoxicity includes clinical examination, ECG, echocardiogram, and serum troponins for any patient who develops hypotension requiring more than one fluid bolus, vasopressors, or transfer to the intensive care unit after ACT treatment [54]. In the most severe cases, requiring constant vasopressor treatment, echocardiogram should be repeated every 2–3 days. Conversely, specific cytokine level measurements are not routinely recommended due to high costs and poor availability.

Management

Management of ACT/CRS-related cardiotoxicity is dependent on the severity of the event. While common measures of cardiac support may be sufficient for mild cases, the most severe cases may require transfer to an intensive care unit and implementation of resuscitative measures, as well as immunosuppressive treatment [54]. The recommended pharmacological treatment of severe ACT-CRS-related cardiotoxicity is tocilizumab, an IL6-receptor antagonist currently approved by the FDA for the treatment of CRS. Corticosteroids can be considered as second-line agents, in particular for those patients not responding to an initial dose of tocilizumab within 24 hours.

Although ACT/CRS-related cardiotoxicity is generally reversible, it can be responsible for fatal outcomes if not recovered. Furthermore, due to the short follow-up assessment currently available, long-term consequences are yet to be elucidated, in particular in view of the long persistence of genetically modified T cells in patients treated with ACT.

Baseline Assessment and General Principle of Management for Cardiovascular IRAE

Due to the low incidence of cardiovascular irAE, few data are available about the optimal cardiovascular assessment before, during, and after immune-therapy. All physicians have to keep in mind that IT can affect the cardiovascular system with a range of different cardiovascular (CV) irAE (Fig. 9.1). Based on high mortality related to immune-related cardiovascular toxicities, a careful evaluation of patients is recommended, including CV-anamnesis and clinical examination before starting IT. Moreover, it might be useful to perform an ECG, echocardiogram, and cardiac biomarkers (troponin and PRO-BNP) as a baseline assessment to permit a comparison during the surveillance phase. When, during IT, a new symptom such as dyspnea, chest pain, palpitation, or syncope appears, a new valuation must be done and compared with basal assessments if available. If a CV irAE is suspected, IT has to be withheld, and immunosuppression therapy should be promptly started. A collaboration between an oncologist and a cardiologist is needful to guarantee the best management and outcome of these toxicities. (Fig. 9.4).

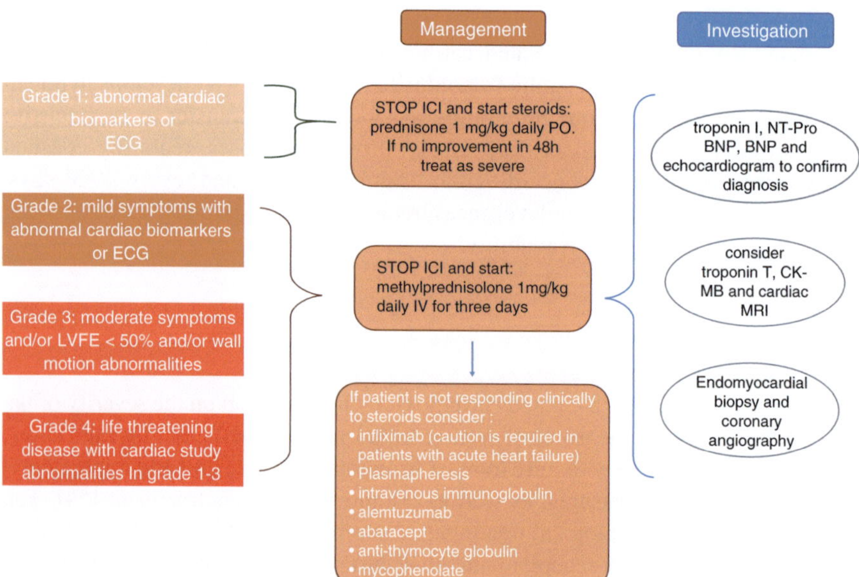

Fig. 9.4 General algorithm for the management of cardiovascular immune-related adverse events

Conclusion

In the complex landscape of new drug development in the immune-oncology field, an adequate comprehension of possible related adverse effects is essential. Cardiotoxicity related to immunotherapy is very rare but potentially fatal. Thus, a deeper understanding of cardiovascular irAEs represents a medical need in this field. An early diagnosis and treatment are indispensable to reverse toxicity when possible. Considering the lack of prospective studies, future research is warranted to understand specific physiopathology mechanism of cardiac irAEs, to establish appropriate monitoring pre- and posttreatment, and to standardize treatment for each different cardiovascular irAEs. The optimal management of patients with cardiovascular irAEs always urges a cooperation between an oncologist and an cardiologist, hopefully in a specialized cardio-oncology unit, to make adequate clinical and treatment decisions and finally improve outcomes.

References

1. Mittal D, Gubin MM, Schreiber RD, Smyth MJ. New insights into cancer immunoediting and its three component phases--elimination, equilibrium and escape. Curr Opin Immunol. 2014;27:16–25.
2. Hanahan D, Weinberg AD. Hallmarks of cancer: the next generation. Cell. 2011;144:646–74.
3. Topalian SL, Hodi FS, Brahmer JR, et al. Safety, activity, and immune correlates of anti-PD-1 antibody in cancer. N Engl J Med. 2012;366:2443–54.
4. Puzanov I, Diab A, Abdallah K, et al. Managing toxicities associated with immune checkpoint inhibitors: consensus recommendations from the Society for Immunotherapy of Cancer (SITC) Toxicity Management Working Group. J Immunother Cancer. 2017;5(1):95.
5. Johnson DB, Balko JM, Compton ML, et al. Fulminant myocarditis with combination immune checkpoint blockade. N Engl J Med. 2016;375(18):1749–55.
6. Salem JE, Manouchehri A, Moey M, et al. Cardiovascular toxicities associated with immune checkpoint inhibitors: an observational retrospective, pharmacovigilance study. Lancet Oncol. 2018;19((12)):1579–89.
7. Mahmood SS, Fradley MG, Cohen JV, et al. Myocarditis in patients treated with immune checkpoint inhibitors. J Am Coll Cardiol. 2018;71((16)):1755–64.
8. Moslehi JJ, Salem JE, Sosman JA, et al. Increased reporting of fatal immune checkpoint inhibitor-associated myocarditis. Lancet. 2018;391(10124):933.
9. Escudier M, Cautela J, Malissen N, et al. Clinical features, management, and outcomes of immune checkpoint inhibitor-related cardiotoxicity. Circulation. 2017;136(21):2085–7.
10. Larkin J, Chiarion-Sileni V, Gonzalez R, et al. Combined nivolumab and ipilimumab or monotherapy in untreated melanoma [published correction appears in N Engl J Med. 2018 Nov 29;379(22):2185]. N Engl J Med. 2015;373(1):23–34.
11. Hu JR, Florido R, Lipson EJ, et al. Cardiovascular toxicities associated with immune checkpoint inhibitors. Cardiovasc Res. 2019;115(5):854–68.
12. Nicolò E, Zagami P, Curigliano G. Antibody-drug conjugates in breast cancer: the chemotherapy of the future? Curr Opin Oncol. 2020;32(5):494–502.
13. Trapani D, Zagami P, Nicolò E, et al. Management of cardiac toxicity induced by chemotherapy. J Clin Med. 2020;9:2885.
14. Okazaki T, Tanaka Y, Nishio R, et al. Autoantibodies against cardiac troponin I are responsible for dilated cardiomyopathy in PD-1-deficient mice. Nat Med. 2003;9:1477–83.

15. Love VA, Grabie N, Duramad P, et al. CTLA4 ablation and interleukin-12 driven differentiation synergistically augment cardiac pathogenicity of cytotoxic T lymphocytes. Circ Res. 2007;101:248–57.
16. Altan M, Toki MI, Gettinger SN, Rimm DL, et al. Immune checkpoint inhibitor–associated pericarditis. J Thorac Oncol. 2019;14:1102–8.
17. Lyon AR, Yousaf N, Battisti NML, et al. Immune checkpoint inhibitors and cardiovascular toxicity. Lancet Oncol. 2018;19(9):e447–58.
18. Wang DY, Salem JE, Cohen JV, et al. Fatal toxic effects associated with immune checkpoint inhibitors: a systematic review and meta-analysis. JAMA Oncol. 2018;4:1721–8.
19. Palaskas N, Lopez-Mattei J, Durand JB, et al. Immune checkpoint inhibitor myocarditis: pathophysiological characteristics, diagnosis, and treatment. J Am Heart Assoc. 2020;9(2):e013757.
20. Nishimura H, Okazaki T, Tanaka Y, et al. Autoimmune dilated cardiomyopathy in PD-1 receptor-deficient mice. Science (80-). 2001;291:319–22.
21. Tivol EA, Borriello F, Schweitzer AN, et al. Loss of CTLA-4 leads to massive lymphoproliferation and fatal multiorgan tissue destruction, revealing a critical negative regulatory role of CTLA-4. Immunity. 1995;3:541–7.
22. Baban B, Liu JY, Qin X, et al. Upregulation of programmed death-1 and its ligand in cardiac injury models: interaction with GADD153. PLoS One. 2015;10:e0124059.
23. Bonaca MP, Olenchock BA, Salem J-E, et al. Myocarditis in the setting of cancer therapeutics. Circulation. 2019;140:80–91.
24. Ferreira VM, Schulz-Menger J, Holmvang G, et al. Cardiovascular magnetic resonance in nonischemic myocardial inflammation: expert recommendations. J Am Coll Cardiol. 2018;72:3158–76.
25. Thomas Aretz H. Myocarditis: the Dallas criteria.1987. Hum Pathol. 1987;18:619–24.
26. Curigliano G, Lenihan D, Fradley M, et al. Management of cardiac disease in cancer patients throughout oncological treatment: ESMO consensus recommendations behalf of the ESMO Guidelines Committee. 2020.
27. Brahmer JR, Lacchetti C, Schneider BJ, et al. Management of immune-related adverse events in patients treated with immune checkpoint inhibitor therapy: American Society of Clinical Oncology Clinical Practice Guideline. J Clin Oncol. 2018;36:1714–68.
28. Thompson JA, Schneider BJ, Brahmer J, et al. Management of Immunotherapy-Related Toxicities, Version 1.2019. J Natl Compr Canc Netw. 2019;17(3):255–89. https://doi.org/10.6004/jnccn.2019.0013. PMID: 30865922.
29. Cancer Institute N Common Terminology Criteria for Adverse Events (CTCAE) Common Terminology Criteria for Adverse Events (CTCAE) v5.0.2017.
30. Hill AB. The environment and disease: association or causation? J R Soc Med. 1965;58:295–300.
31. Du S, Zhou L, Alexander GS, et al. PD-1 modulates radiation-induced cardiac toxicity through cytotoxic T lymphocytes. J Thorac Oncol. 2018;13:510–20.
32. Adler Y, Charron P, Imazio M, et al. ESC guidelines for the diagnosis and management of pericardial diseases.2015. Eur Heart J. 2015;36:2921–64.
33. Chahine J, Collier P, Maroo A, et al. Myocardial and pericardial toxicity associated with immune checkpoint inhibitors in cancer patients. JACC Case Rep. 2020;2:191–9.
34. Ferreira M, Pichon E, Carmier D, et al. Coronary toxicities of anti-PD-1 and anti-PD-L1 immunotherapies: a case report and review of the literature and international registries. Target Oncol. 2018;13(4):509–15.
35. Hu YB, Zhang Q, Li HJ, et al. Evaluation of rare but severe immune related adverse effects meta-analysis. Transl Lung Cancer Res. 2017;6:s8–20.
36. Bazaz R, Marriott HM, Francis SE, Dockrell DH. Mechanistic links between acute respiratory tract infections and acute coronary syndromes. J Infect. 2013;66:1e17.
37. Nykl R, Fischer O, Vykoupil K, Taborsky M. A unique reason for coronary spasm causing temporary ST elevation myocardial infarction (inferior STEMI) – systemic inflammatory response syndrome after use of pembrolizumab. Arch Med Sci Atheroscler Dis. 2017;2:e100e2.

38. Amsterdam EA, Wenger NK, Brindis RG, et al. 2014 AHA/ACC guideline for the management of patients with non-ST-elevation acute coronary syndromes: a report of the American College of Cardiology/American Heart Association Task Force on Practice Guidelines. Circulation. 2014;130:e344e426.

39. Roffi M, Patrono C, Collet JP, et al. 2015 ESC guidelines for the management of acute coronary syndromes in patients presenting without persistent ST-segment elevation. Task force for the management of acute coronary syndromes in patients presenting without persistent ST-segment elevation of the European society of cardiology (ESC). G Ital Cardiol (Rome). 2016;17:831e72.

40. Chen DY, Huang WK, Chien-Chia Wu V, et al. Cardiovascular toxicity of immune checkpoint inhibitors in cancer patients: A review when cardiology meets immuno-oncology. J Formos Med Assoc. 2020;119(10):1461–75. https://doi.org/10.1016/j.jfma.2019.07.025. Epub 2019 Aug 20. PMID: 31444018.

41. Cardiovascular toxicity of immune checkpoint inhibitors in cancer patients: a review when cardiology meets immuno-oncology. J Formos Med Assoc. 2019;S0929–6646(19)30408–5.

42. Lyon AR, Bossone E, Schneider B, et al. Current state of knowledge on Takotsubo syndrome: a position statement from the taskforce on Takotsubo syndrome of the heart failure Association of the European Society of Cardiology. Eur J Heart Fail. 2016;18:8–26.

43. Ederhy S, Cautela J, Ancedy Y, et al. Takotsubo-like syndrome in cancer patients treated with immune checkpoint inhibitors. JACC Cardiovasc Imaging. 2018;11(8):1187–90.

44. Lopez EM, Dunn S, Mazimba S. Malignant arrhythmias in autoimmune myocarditis secondary to immune checkpoint blockade treatment. J Am Coll Cardiol. 2018;71(11):A2375.

45. Tajiri K, Ieda M. Cardiac complications in immune checkpoint inhibition therapy. Front Cardiovasc Med 2019;6.

46. Kamesh L, Heward JM, Williams JM, et al. CT60 and +49 polymorphisms of CTLA 4 are associated with ANCA-positive small vessel vasculitis. Rheumatology. 2009;48(12):1502–5.

47. Boland P, Heath J, Sandigursky S. Immune checkpoint inhibitors and vasculitis. Curr Opin Rheumatol. 2020;32(1):53–6.

48. Daxini A, Cronin K, Sreih AG. Vasculitis associated with immune checkpoint inhibitors—a systematic review. Clin Rheumatol. 2018;37(9):2579–84.

49. Eleftheriou D, Brogan PA. Therapeutic advances in the treatment of vasculitis. Pediatr Rheumatol. 2016;14(1):26.

50. Wolf B, Zimmermann S, Arber C, Irving M, Trueb L, Coukos G. Safety and tolerability of adoptive cell therapy in cancer. Drug Saf. 2019;42(2):315–34.

51. Lee DW, Kochenderfer JN, Stetler-Stevenson M, et al. T cells expressing CD19 chimeric antigen receptors for acute lymphoblastic leukaemia in children and young adults: a phase 1 dose-escalation trial. Lancet. 2015;385(9967):517–28.

52. Kochenderfer JN, Dudley ME, Kassim SH, et al. Chemotherapy-refractory diffuse large B-cell lymphoma and indolent B-cell malignancies can be effectively treated with autologous T cells expressing an anti-CD19 chimeric antigen receptor. J Clin Oncol. 2015;33(6):540–9.

53. Linette GP, Stadtmauer EA, Maus MV, et al. Cardiovascular toxicity and titin cross-reactivity of affinity-enhanced T cells in myeloma and melanoma. Blood. 2013;122(6):863–71.

54. Brudno JN, Kochenderfer JN. Toxicities of chimeric antigen receptor T cells: recognition and management. Blood. 2016;127(26):3321–30.

Future Perspectives

10

Dimitrios Farmakis

Introduction

Cancer and cardiovascular (CV) diseases represent the two leading causes of mortality. Importantly, these two conditions interact, affecting the management and worsening the prognosis of each other. In addition, cancer may increase the incidence of CV disease through its direct and indirect effects on the heart and vessels and most importantly through the CV toxicity of anticancer therapies. The importance of CV health and outcomes in patients with cancer becomes increasingly important as the advances in anticancer therapies lead to a continuous improvement in patients' survival.

The intersection between CV disease and cancer represents the objective of cardio-oncology, a new but rapidly evolving field of cardiovascular medicine. The rapid increase in the clinical and research efforts in this field is depicted by the growing number of dedicated cardio-oncology clinics and services throughout the world and the rapidly accumulating relevant publications over the past few years. This rapid development of the field is driven mostly by the clinical needs imposed by the increasing survival of cancer patients, on the one hand, and the evolving complexity of anticancer modalities that are often followed by CV adverse events, on the other [1]. However, this rapid growth leads inevitably to many unanswered questions that need to be addressed by future research. The scope of this chapter is to outline the main challenges and perspectives in the field of cardio-oncology, covering basic, translational, and clinical research, education and training, and service organization and provision.

D. Farmakis (✉)
University of Cyprus Medical School, Nicosia, Cyprus
e-mail: farmakis.dimitrios@ucy.ac.cy

A. Russo et al. (eds.), *Cardio-Oncology*, Current Clinical Pathology,
https://doi.org/10.1007/978-3-030-97744-3_10

Basic and Translational Research

Cancer is known to cause heart disease through the toxicity of anticancer therapies, covered extensively in this chapter, the invasion of the heart and vessels, and the activation of a systemic inflammatory and wasting process [2]. In addition, it has been proposed that specific cancer byproducts may exert a direct cardiotoxic effect, affecting cardiac function [3]. On the other hand, preliminary evidence shows that the diseased heart releases in the circulation substances that may act as mediators of oncogenesis that may facilitate cancer development [4]. Regardless of the potential reciprocal pathogenetic association between cancer and CV disease, the two conditions share several common risk factors that predispose to both, including ageing, smoking, obesity, physical inactivity, and cardiometabolic factors and comorbidities [5]. Besides risk factors, common pathogenetic pathways, such as clonal hematopoiesis, may lead to the parallel development of CV disease and cancer [3]. The delineation of this reciprocal relationship with the identification of the implicated mediators, pathways, and processes represents currently a growing field of research.

Clinical Research

Our knowledge of cardiotoxicity and its timely diagnosis, prevention, and management is currently accumulating rapidly as indicated by the exponential increase in the number of published papers in the field. As new effective anticancer drugs are entering the clinical arena, new cardiotoxicity profiles are being discovered. This has been particularly true for the innovative immunotherapies that have emerged over the past few years as very promising anticancer modalities. The risk of myocarditis, among other immune-mediated adverse events, associated with immune checkpoint inhibitors, has only recently been identified following the increasing use of these drugs for the treatment of several malignancies [6]. Similarly, chimeric antigen receptor (CAR) T-cell therapy, another form of immunotherapy, is currently being studied for its cardiotoxicity profile, as it has been found to induce arrhythmias, hemodynamic compromise, and cardiac dysfunction as part of a profound systemic cytokine release syndrome [7]. As long as new anticancer agents are being introduced in clinical practice, the investigation for cardiotoxicity will continue.

The optimal integration of accumulated knowledge in clinical practice and its transformation into clinical management protocols and guidelines remains an important challenge. Three specific aspects are relevant in this regard: (i) the baseline stratification of the risk of cardiotoxicity based on history, risk factors, and clinical findings that would further delineate the need and intensity of monitoring during and after cancer therapy; (ii) the optimal use of sensitive biomarkers and imaging techniques for the monitoring and timely diagnosis of early cardiotoxicity in terms of choice and timing (in other words, what to measure and when); and (iii)

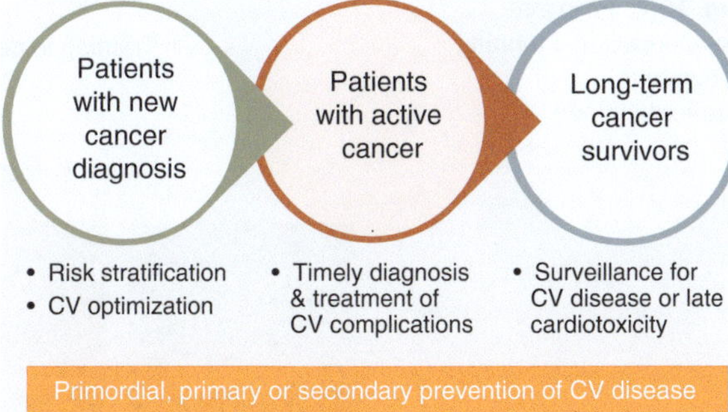

Fig. 10.1 Components of a structured cardio-oncology program or service

the application of primary prevention interventions based on the findings of baseline risk stratification and monitoring modalities (Fig. 10.1). In this context, the Heart Failure Association of the European Society of Cardiology has produced a series of position papers summarizing the current knowledge on baseline risk stratification and the role of biomarkers and cardiac imaging in the assessment and monitoring of cancer patients that may serve as a base for clinical practice and future research. A tailored approach to the management of cancer patients in terms of CV monitoring modalities, follow-up intervals, CV treatments, and therapeutic decisions regarding anticancer drugs is essential [8]. This need renders cardio-oncology an evolving field of precision medicine [1].

Education and Training

The CV evaluation and management of patients with cancer requires a combination of expertise and clinical skills in the diagnosis and management of CV disease along with sufficient knowledge of cancer and its therapy. As a result, a general cardiologist or a cardiologist sub-specialist requires additional training to organize and deliver a cardio-oncology service.

Current education and training of CV physicians in cardio-oncology is performed mainly through special sessions in congresses, dedicated seminars, established fellowships, and structured courses. A training course would ideally provide comprehensive theoretical and practical training on cardio-oncology that would equip the trainees with the necessary theoretical and practical knowledge so they are able to deliver a cardio-oncology service. The development of a dedicated cardio-oncology course requires the delineation of a common cardio-oncology curriculum approved by international scientific associations and local authorities as well as the establishment of processes of accreditation and certification of training centers and graduates (Fig. 10.2). The ensuing step could be the recognition of cardio-oncology as an official sub-specialty of cardiovascular medicine.

Fig. 10.2 Proposed
components of a training
program in
cardio-oncology

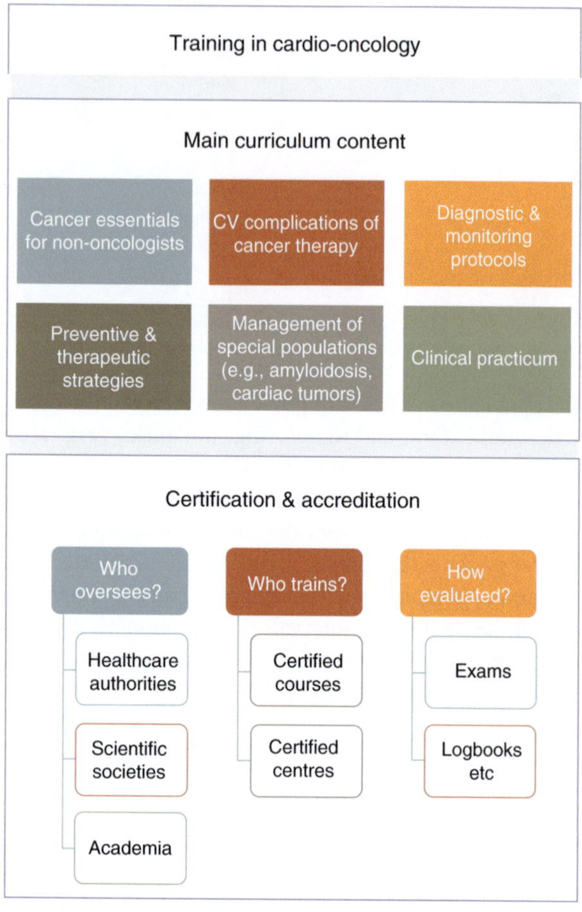

Service Organization and Provision

Besides being a dynamic field of basic, translational, and clinical research, there is a continuously rising demand for cardio-oncology services due to the increasing number of cancer patients and survivors, the evolving complexity of anticancer therapies, and the growing impact of CV disease on these patients [1]. An effective cardio-oncology service renders the majority of cancer patients fit to receive the best available anticancer treatment without compromises or interruptions because of CV issues, thus contributing to the improved management and outcomes of these patients [8, 9].

A series of steps have been proposed for the organization of an effective cardio-oncology service (Fig. 10.3). The main steps concern the population of the service with adequately trained healthcare professionals, the precise definition of the provided services, the development of specific criteria for patients' referral to the service, the definition of general monitoring and treatment protocols, which should always be individualized to each patient's characteristics, and, last but not least, the

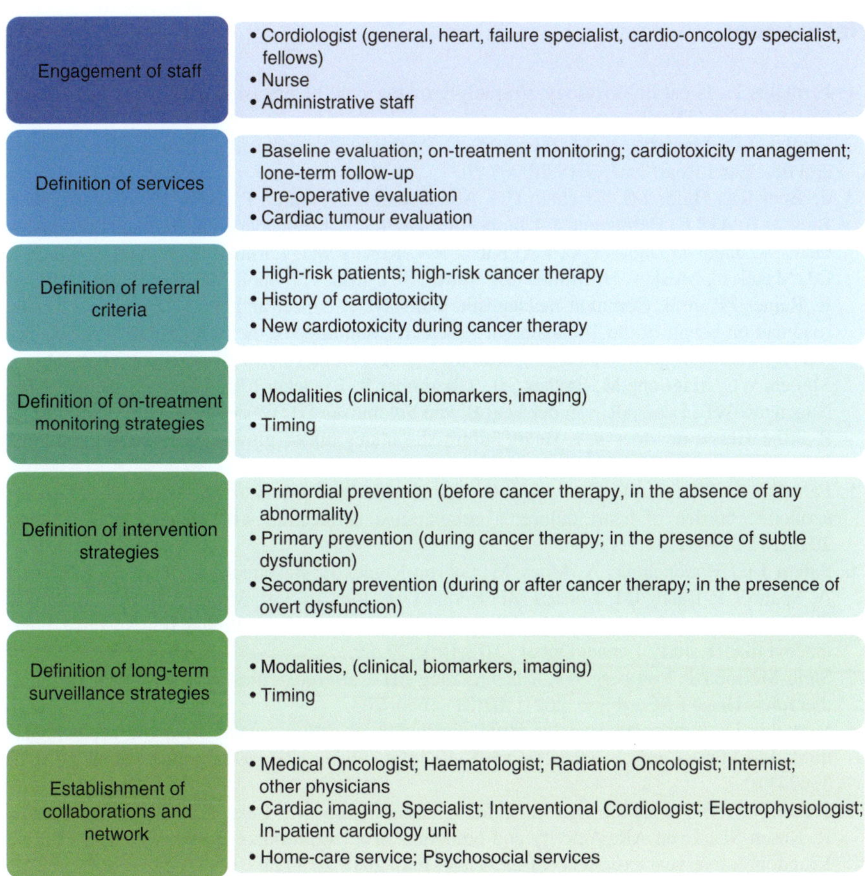

Fig. 10.3 Steps for the development of an effective cardio-oncology service. (Reprinted with permission from Farmakis et al. [10])

establishment of effective collaboration and networking among implicated health-care professionals and clinics [10]. These steps should be based on some general principles that govern the CV assessment and management of cancer patients, delineated by guidelines, position statements, and other documents [11], but should further be tailored to the local infrastructures, available manpower and resources, and clinical needs. Such an approach would allow the effective integration of the cardio-oncology service within the existing healthcare infrastructures and would further facilitate the establishment of a functional patient pathway through the implicated services and the development of proper collaboration and communication among the implicated healthcare professionals. In addition, integration of individual clinics into greater regional, national, and international cardio-oncology networks is required to facilitate clinical and research collaboration and allow the generation of epidemiological evidence that would further enable the better organization of provided services [12].

References

1. Farmakis D. Is cardio-oncology a rapidly growing field of precision medicine? Eur J Heart Fail. 2020;22:2310–3.
2. Farmakis D, Mantzourani M, Filippatos G. Anthracycline-induced cardiomyopathy: secrets and lies. Eur J Heart Fail. 2018;20:907–9.
3. de Boer RA, Hulot J-S, Tocchetti CG, Aboumsallem JP, Ameri P, Anker SD, Bauersachs J, Bertero E, AJS C, Čelutkienė J, Chioncel O, Dodion P, Eschenhagen T, Farmakis D, Bayes-Genis A, Jäger D, Jankowska EA, Kitsis RN, Konety SH, Larkin J, Lehmann L, Lenihan DJ, Maack C, Moslehi JJ, Müller OJ, Nowak-Sliwinska P, Piepoli MF, Ponikowski P, Pudil R, Rainer PP, et al. Common mechanistic pathways in cancer and heart failure. A scientific roadmap on behalf of the Translational Research Committee of the Heart Failure Association (HFA) of the European Society of Cardiology (ESC). Eur J Heart Fail. 2020;22:2272–89.
4. Meijers WC, Maglione M, Bakker SJL, Oberhuber R, Kieneker LM, de Jong S, Haubner BJ, Nagengast WB, Lyon AR, van der Vegt B, van Veldhuisen DJ, Westenbrink BD, van der Meer P, Silljé HHW, de Boer RA. Heart failure stimulates tumor growth by circulating factors. Circulation. 2018;138:678–91.
5. Farmakis D, Stafylas P, Giamouzis G, Maniadakis N, Parissis J. The medical and socio-economic burden of heart failure: a comparative delineation with cancer. Int J Cardiol. 2016;203:279–81.
6. Salem J-E, Manouchehri A, Moey M, Lebrun-Vignes B, Bastarache L, Pariente A, Gobert A, Spano J-P, Balko JM, Bonaca MP, Roden DM, Johnson DB, Moslehi JJ. Cardiovascular toxicities associated with immune checkpoint inhibitors: an observational, retrospective, pharmacovigilance study. Lancet Oncol. 2018;19:1579–89.
7. Stein-Merlob AF, Rothberg MV, Ribas A, Yang EH. Cardiotoxicities of novel cancer immuno-therapies. Heart Br Card Soc. 2021;107(21):1694–703.
8. Farmakis D. Anticoagulation for atrial fibrillation in active cancer: what the cardiologists think. Eur J Prev Cardiol. 2021;28(6):608–10. https://doi.org/10.1093/eurjpc/zwaa087. PMID: 33624110.
9. Pareek N, Cevallos J, Moliner P, Shah M, Tan LL, Chambers V, Baksi AJ, Khattar RS, Sharma R, Rosen SD, Lyon AR. Activity and outcomes of a cardio-oncology service in the United Kingdom-a five-year experience. Eur J Heart Fail. 2018;20:1721–31.
10. Farmakis D, Keramida K, Filippatos G. How to build a cardio-oncology service? Eur J Heart Fail. 2018;20:1732–4.
11. Zamorano JL, Lancellotti P, Rodriguez Muñoz D, Aboyans V, Asteggiano R, Galderisi M, Habib G, Lenihan DJ, Lip GYH, Lyon AR, Lopez Fernandez T, Mohty D, Piepoli MF, Tamargo J, Torbicki A, Suter TM, Zamorano JL, Aboyans V, Achenbach S, Agewall S, Badimon L, Barón-Esquivias G, Baumgartner H, Bax JJ, Bueno H, Carerj S, Dean V, Erol Ç, Fitzsimons D, Gaemperli O, et al. 2016 ESC Position Paper on cancer treatments and cardiovascular toxicity developed under the auspices of the ESC Committee for Practice Guidelines: The Task Force for cancer treatments and cardiovascular toxicity of the European Society of Cardiology (ESC). Eur J Heart Fail. 2017;19:9–42.
12. Taskforce of the Hellenic Heart Failure Clinics Network. Distribution, infrastructure, and expertise of heart failure and cardio-oncology clinics in a developing network: temporal evolution and challenges during the coronavirus disease 2019 pandemic. ESC Heart Fail. 2020;7:3408–13.

Index

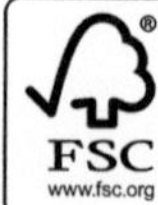

MIX
Papier aus verantwortungsvollen Quellen
Paper from responsible sources
FSC® C105338

If you have any concerns about our products,
you can contact us on
ProductSafety@springernature.com

In case Publisher is established outside the EU,
the EU authorized representative is:
Springer Nature Customer Service Center GmbH
Europaplatz 3, 69115 Heidelberg, Germany

Printed by Libri Plureos GmbH
in Hamburg, Germany